Oct. 7, 2009

P9-BYN-326

BRANCH

WITHDRAWN

THE EVERYTHING® GUIDE TO BEING VEGETARIAN

Dear Reader,

As with any cookbook undertaking, the challenge is to find a way to present information and introduce recipes that will entice readers into the kitchen. For both longtime and novice vegetarians, getting the facts straight is key. But also learning about what can go into the cookpot besides the soyfood and bean staples will provide years of great cooking and eating. To these ends, an author's challenge today is to know when to stop writing about all the exciting ingredients that are available. Why? Because the marketplace is now brimming with a cornucopia of ingredients, all basics for building sound meals by imparting diverse flavors and textures. With modern technology, of course, our globe and our markets have shrunk, and it's very easy to infuse flavors from every cuisine around the world. That's what makes cooking and eating such an exciting life adventure! So, for everyone who wants to build better health, head to the kitchen and start cooking.

Alexandra Greeley

Welcome to the EVERYTHING® Series!

These handy, accessible books give you all you need to tackle a difficult project, gain a new hobby, comprehend a fascinating topic, prepare for an exam, or even brush up on something you learned back in school but have since forgotten.

You can choose to read an *Everything*® book from cover to cover or just pick out the information you want from our four useful boxes: e-questions, e-facts, e-alerts, and e-ssentials.

We give you everything you need to know on the subject, but throw in a lot of fun stuff along the way, too.

We now have more than 400 *Everything*® books in print, spanning such wide-ranging categories as weddings, pregnancy, cooking, music instruction, foreign language, crafts, pets, New Age, and so much more. When you're done reading them all, you can finally say you know *Everything*®!

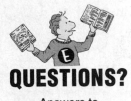

QUESTIONS?
Answers to
common questions

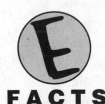

FACTS
Important snippets
of information

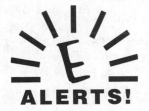

ALERTS!
Urgent
warnings

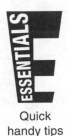

ESSENTIALS
Quick
handy tips

PUBLISHER Karen Cooper

DIRECTOR OF ACQUISITIONS AND INNOVATION Paula Munier

MANAGING EDITOR, EVERYTHING SERIES Lisa Laing

COPY CHIEF Casey Ebert

ACQUISITIONS EDITOR Katie McDonough/Katrina Schroeder

DEVELOPMENT EDITOR Brett Palana-Shanahan

EDITORIAL ASSISTANT Hillary Thompson

Visit the entire Everything® series at *www.everything.com*

THE
EVERYTHING®
GUIDE TO BEING VEGETARIAN

613.242
GRE

The advice, nutrition information, and recipes you need to enjoy a healthy lifestyle

Alexandra Greeley

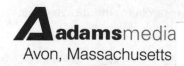

Avon, Massachusetts

Algonquin Area Public Library
Eastgate Branch
115 Eastgate Drive
Algonquin, IL 60102

To my children and their families, so they may always enjoy the
fruits—and grains and vegetables—of nature's bounty.

Copyright © 2009 by F+W Media, Inc.
All rights reserved.
This book, or parts thereof, may not be reproduced
in any form without permission from the publisher; exceptions
are made for brief excerpts used in published reviews.

An Everything® Series Book.
Everything® and everything.com® are registered trademarks of F+W Media, Inc.

Published by Adams Media, a division of F+W Media, Inc.
57 Littlefield Street, Avon, MA 02322 U.S.A.
www.adamsmedia.com

ISBN 10: 1-60550-051-8
ISBN 13: 978-1-60550-051-5

Printed in the United States of America.

J   I   H   G   F   E   D   C   B   A

Library of Congress Cataloging-in-Publication Data
is available from the publisher.

his publication is designed to provide accurate and authoritative information with regard to the subject matter covered. It is sold with the understanding that the publisher is not engaged in rendering legal, accounting, or other professional advice. If legal advice or other expert assistance is required, the services of a competent professional person should be sought.

—From a *Declaration of Principles* jointly adopted by a Committee of the American Bar Association and a Committee of Publishers and Associations

Many of the designations used by manufacturers and sellers to distinguish their products are claimed as trademarks. Where those designations appear in this book and Adams Media was aware of a trademark claim, the designations have been printed with initial capital letters.

This book is available at quantity discounts for bulk purchases.
For information, please call 1-800-289-0963.

Contents

Acknowledgments

I thank all the numerous voices on the other end of phone lines or respondents who answered e-mails. They have shared their vegetarian and other wisdom, helping to sort out fact from fiction. In particular, special thanks to John Cunningham and Reed Mangels of the Vegetarian Resource Group, in Baltimore, Maryland; a spokesman for the National Pasta Association in Washington, D.C.; Katherine Tallmadge, spokesperson for the American Dietetic Association and president of Personalized Nutrition, in Washington, D.C.; the Nemours Foundation's Center for Children's Health Media, corporate headquarters in Jacksonville, Florida; and the staff at the Soyfoods Association of North America in Washington, D.C.

A word of gratitude to some family members, especially to my daughter, Susan, for tasting comments and eating so many tested recipes; my son, Dr. Christopher, for pediatric input; my son, Michael, for continued interest and support; and my sister, Mary Hager, for insightful content comments.

And finally, a thank-you to my agent, Robert Diforio, who started this all.

Top Ten Health Benefits to Being a Vegetarian

1. Vegetarians are less likely to become obese.

2. Vegetarians are less likely to develop coronary heart disease.

3. Vegetarians are less likely to develop high blood pressure.

4. Vegetarians are less likely to develop diabetes.

5. Vegetarians are less likely to suffer from certain cancers.

6. Vegetarians may develop less osteoporosis.

7. Vegetarians may suffer less from constipation.

8. Vegetarians may develop fewer gallstones.

9. Vegetarians are more likely to feel better and stay slimmer.

10. Vegetarians are likely to live longer.

Introduction

▶TO MAINSTREAM AMERICA, vegetarianism may seem mysterious and perhaps even cultlike, a way of living probably associated with the hippie communes of decades past. But judging by the growing numbers of people who are choosing a plant-based diet over one that includes eating flesh and animal products, the ideals of vegetarianism are becoming more appealing. The reason is that the more people understand the movement, the more it can make good, plain sense.

Embracing the vegetarian lifestyle can be very straightforward: Just omit all meats, meat products, and seafood from your diet, and then carefully select menus filled with vegetables, fruit, legumes, dairy products, and whole grains. Together these should meet your dietary needs. Sounds simple, and it is. After all, generations of folks here and around the world have made that choice and lived the life—and thrived and prospered.

But the reasons for selecting vegetarianism can be varied—and can also be very complex. For some with weight or coronary problems, vegetarianism may be a big part of the solution. For others, it's a matter of conscience or morality, and of respecting the right to life of all living creatures, whether they walk, crawl, slither, fly, or swim. And for still other people, vegetarianism is a key part of their religious life, proscribed by the dictates of their faith. Take practicing Chinese Buddhists, for example, who are forbidden to kill or to eat flesh. And Chinese vegetarian restaurants, usually affiliated with a Buddhist temple, serve very highly refined vegetarian dishes, many of which, ironically, resemble meat. Closer to home in the United States, many Seventh

Day Adventists practice vegetarianism, and many inside and outside their faith believe that their dietary habits, plus their abstention from alcohol and tobacco, contribute to their noteworthy longevity.

No matter whether you decide to adopt the vegetarian way of eating wholly or partially, you should know that selecting vegetarian options and preparing all-veg meals have become much easier than ever before. Not only can you find good vegetarian restaurants in almost every city, but also most restaurant menus offer at least one vegetarian entrée, and certainly, a responsible chef who aims to please customers will cook an all-veg dish to order. Most supermarkets and certainly all health food stores stock a plethora of vegetarian ingredients, from soymilks and soy-based products to whole grains, greens, and fruits. Even the burgeoning growth of farmers' markets across the American landscape provides a valuable resource for people looking for a healthful, natural way to stock their pantries and refrigerators.

The best part for home cooks is this: vegetarian recipes have merged into the modern age, shedding the image that meals are based on tasteless grains-and-greens combos with just a dollop of bland tofu. Cookbooks have compiled countless enticing dishes that bring together the best of ethnic cooking plus the most creative ways to use today's ingredients. In the past, who would have guessed you could prepare a meal that might feature Turkish-style stuffed peppers using a soy meat substitute or one that pairs field greens and goat cheese for a rich quiche? In fact, modern vegetarians can travel the globe or create a whole new entrée without leaving town.

On another note, most vegetarians have come to realize they are not alone in making this lifestyle choice. Based on the 2007 Census Bureau report numbering the population at 301 million people, the total number of Americans who are vegetarian would be about 7.5 million. And that group of people has fostered the growth of a vegetarian-lifestyle industry: social groups, singles groups, dating clubs, and travel groups, to name a few of the vegetarian activities. So if you are considering making the change, you might flip through your yellow pages, contact such groups as the Vegetarian Resource Group at *www.vrg.org*, or check out *www.TheVegetarianSite.com* to find out more about the vegetarian lifestyle.

CHAPTER 1

What Does "Vegetarian" Really Mean?

For anyone who has tuned into the national dialogues about the environment or about eating for good health, the term *vegetarian* must certainly be familiar. Even so, precisely what that means causes plenty of confusion. Some "vegetarians" continue to eat chicken; others include seafood. Still others exempt all meat and dairy products from their kitchen. So just what is a vegetarian?

Defining the Term and the Movement

According to the United States Department of Agriculture (USDA), a vegetarian is someone who primarily eats a plant-based diet. That's the simple definition, but vegetarianism encompasses many different lifestyles and interpretations of just what a plant-based diet is. For example, vegans are really vegetarians-plus, for they exclude from their diet all animal products—including dairy goods and eggs—and refuse to use any animal byproducts, including wool, leather, and silk.

What Is a Vegetarian?

What vegetarians have in common is that they stick to an eating plan that has been solidly endorsed by the American Dietetic Association (ADA) as healthful and nutritious when properly planned. Further, the ADA states that the health benefits of a vegetarian diet may help to prevent or treat a host of chronic problems, from obesity to high blood pressure, so long as the diet is balanced and includes a wide range of nonmeat ingredients.

As with any diet, then, mapping out the right eating plan is at the top of the must-do list. That's especially important for adults making the switch to a no-meat diet who have depended on getting proteins from their daily meat servings. It's easy to think in terms of heaping portions of steamed vegetables and bowls of sweet fruit, but adding good protein sources to a week's menu takes knowledge about food basics.

Defining the Movement

Today's vegetarian movement is not an outgrowth of twentieth-century political or social movements, for vegetarianism may be as old as mankind. But the movement received its modern-day moniker in the nineteenth century, when the British Vegetarian Society used the phrase "vegetarian" to describe those who followed a plant-based diet. It's possible that the term itself was derived from the Latin word *vegetus*, meaning "lively" or "strong," though not every historian agrees with that. In any case, the fact remains: vegetarians eat vegetables and other plant-derived foods.

Who Are Vegetarians?

Vegetarians may come from any walk of life, from any educational background, from any culture, and from any age group. So the word "vegetarian" really describes a diverse group of people.

Vegetarian Diets

Eating plants as food is basic to all vegetarians, but over time people have devised many different vegetarian categories to suit their various beliefs and lifestyles. For beginners, the distinctions may seem bewildering.

- **Lacto-Ovó:** Perhaps the largest group, these vegetarians eat both dairy products and eggs, but no meat of any kind. Their food plan is broad and offers substantial choices to include greens, grains, fruits, and legumes, plus moderate amounts of nuts, dairy products, eggs, and plant oils, and in the smallest quantities, sweets.
- **Lacto:** This group omits eggs but does include all dairy products in a diet that otherwise resembles the lacto-ovó food plan.
- **Ovó:** These vegetarians include eggs but omit all dairy products in a diet that otherwise resembles the typical vegetarian one.
- **Vegan:** Following the strictest plant-based diet, a vegan excludes eating or using all animal meats or products, including all dairy, eggs, and honey. And a strict vegan will not wear anything made from silk, leather, or wool. They are careful to avoid eating any processed foods that may have required animal products in their manufacture, such as refined sugar. While the eating plan sounds restrictive, careful vegans plan their meals to include a wide range of nutrient-dense foods.
- **Flexitarian:** Whether you call this group flexitarian or semi-vegetarian, these people do include some meat in their diet. Some people may eat fish (pescatarian) but no red meat or poultry; for health reasons, this particular form of vegetarianism is increasingly popular. Some may eat poultry, but no red meat or fish. And others may limit their meat intake to an occasional meal. But to the active vegetarian community, flexitarians are just vegetarians in the making.

- **Macrobiotic:** While a macrobiotic diet is not strictly all vegetarian all the time—it may include seafood—it is plant-based, and prohibits the use of refined sugars, dairy products, and nightshade plants such as potatoes and tomatoes. The diet may have Greek roots, but it has an Asian pedigree: its founder, a Japanese doctor, turned to Buddhist and Chinese principles to create a diet that includes many Asian food-stuffs, such as miso, tofu, tempeh, Asian greens, and sea vegetables.
- **Fruitarians:** As the word implies, this group eats mainly fresh raw fruit and nuts and seeds, including sprouts. Believers claim that their diet promotes good health, but because it lacks substantial protein sources, it is not suitable for youngsters. Note that long-term fruitarians may lose a dramatic amount of weight.
- **Raw Foodists:** Most raw foodists are vegans, eating only fruits and vegetables—preferably organic—as they are found in their natural state. But occasionally, some raw foodists eat raw meat and eggs and drink certified raw milk and other certified raw dairy products.

Why Become a Vegetarian?

People turn to vegetarianism for many different and often compelling reasons. For some it's about health; for others, it's about ending animal cruelty. And increasingly, vegetarianism appeals to an activist population concerned about environmental issues.

Health Reasons

With their increased worries about the growing incidence of chronic diseases, many Americans cite health as the reason for changing lifestyle and diet. According to the Centers for Disease Control (CDC), the leading causes of death in the United States are cancer, diabetes, and heart disease, all of which account for about 1.7 million deaths annually. But the sad truth, say the experts at the American Heart Association, American Cancer Society, and others, is that many of these deaths would have been preventable if the patient had altered his or her diet to reduce consumption of saturated fats (animal fats) and had exercised regularly. Vegetarians, particularly vegans, can drastically reduce their fat intake.

Furthermore, research shows that vegetarians are less likely to become obese; to develop coronary heart disease, high blood pressure, or diabetes; or to suffer from certain cancers. Vegetarians may develop less osteoporosis, suffer less often from constipation, and develop fewer gallstones. It's easy to see why many people become vegetarians simply to feel better, stay slimmer, and to possibly live longer.

Ethical Reasons

According to the USDA, the per-capita meat consumption—including red meat, poultry, and seafood—in 2005 totaled about 200 pounds, an amount 22 pounds higher than in 1970. But statistics show that red meat consumption itself has dropped significantly, perhaps reflecting the consumer's growing awareness of animal rights.

Numerous reports of the cruel living conditions of animals on factory farms may account for this drop. But whether you are an animal activist or simply a pet owner, you may abstain from eating meat out of respect for an animal's life. Yet it's important to remember that people in some cultures, such as the Inuit, have traditionally subsisted on a basic diet of fish and meat; other cultures live on a diet consisting of proteins from animals such as snakes and insects.

Religious Beliefs

Numerous religions—including some Buddhist sects, Jains, Hindus, and Seventh Day Adventists—support a plant-based diet, or at least recommend their believers embrace a vegetarian lifestyle. Other religions, such as Judaism and Islam, prohibit eating certain kinds of meat, specifically pork; Jews who keep kosher follow stricter meat-eating laws, for they are forbidden to consume specific animal or animal products or to eat certain fish and shellfish. And many Baha'is prefer following a vegetarian diet because they believe a plant-based diet is how future generations should eat.

Environmentalism

Global warming, the greenhouse effect, and pollution all play a role in how concerned citizens view their shrinking and endangered natural resources. Many consumers now see a link between their health and the planet's health, and are beginning to believe, for example, that supporting livestock on limited agricultural lands just for meat consumption is speeding up the destruction of land and water resources. That is particularly worrisome as populations grow and the demand for meat keeps pace with that growth.

Although these concerns are not new—Frances Moore Lappé wrote about them in 1972 in her seminal book *Diet for a Small Planet*—present-day activist groups such as Greenpeace note that raising animals for food uses up and/or destroys valuable natural resources, including land, water, and the grains used for feeding animals. As they point out, not only do cattle produce quantities of waste requiring treatment, but also farmed animals consume about 70 percent of the grains and cereals American farmers grow each year, an amount that could presumably feed nearly 9 billion people. In those terms, changing to a plant-based diet could make a positive environmental impact—and feed more people.

An Ideal with Historical Roots

Was man's first foods animal or vegetable? Of course, no one knows for sure, but records show that certain Egyptian religious groups followed vegetarian principles based on their ideas of how the souls of the departed might reappear in living creatures, including animals. Thereafter, followers of the ancient Greek mathematician and philosopher Pythagoras (circa 572 to 490 B.C.), who himself spent time in Egypt, followed a vegetarian diet. And ancient (and many modern) Hindus, Zoroastrians, Buddhists, and Jainists—whose basic tenets focused on respect for the lives of all creatures—encouraged others to follow a nonmeat diet. Clearly, vegetarianism has very deep roots in mankind's history.

Vegetarianism's Origins

While vegetarianism in man's earliest eras did not have mainstream acceptance—eating meat was often a sign of one's social status and wealth—it did appeal to various groups throughout history. By the 1600s, the ideals of a vegetarian lifestyle became fashionable among some members of European society, especially those who were becoming influenced by the ideals of humanism. Their exposure to the ideals of Indian vegetarianism—doing no harm to any living creatures—helped to change influential thinkers of the day.

As Tristram Stuart writes in his book *The Bloodless Revolution*, intellectuals and radicals challenged the standards of the day—that slaughtering animals for food was acceptable. These early arguments, Stuart contends, became the impetus for and the founding of today's various vegetarian movements and societies. By the early twentieth century, a group in Europe had founded the International Vegetarian Union (IVU) at the first World Vegetarian Congress in Germany. A nonprofit organization dedicated to promoting vegetarianism worldwide, it holds regular world congresses in different countries.

Vegetarianism in America

It may seem hard to believe, but American vegetarianism was a vital movement long before the 1960s counterculture brought its ideals to light. Dating back to the late 1700s, during the period when new immigrants discovered America's vast natural resources and were shooting buffalo for hides and not for meat, vegetarian ideals were taking hold, if not for philosophical or health reasons, at least for economic ones. Urban dwellers in the nineteenth and early twentieth centuries often found that meat was scarce and expensive—and often unsafe for eating.

What they were discovering, thanks to the discoveries of such health advocates and reformers as the Reverend Sylvester Graham and John Kellogg, was that diets based on grains and the vast array of the New World's fruits and vegetables offered a new and healthful way to eat.

Noteworthy Vegetarians

As you look back over the history of vegetarianism, you may be surprised by how many famous people have given up eating meat—either all or most of the time—and embraced the vegetarian lifestyle. The following notables have been cited as vegetarians, though finding proof is difficult: Greek philosophers Epicurus (whose name has become the moniker for the highest standards of eating, or Epicureanism), Plato, and Plutarch;

Leonardo da Vinci; and America's own Ben Franklin described themselves as vegetarian.

Other contemporary figures who may have been part- or full-time vegetarians include George Bernard Shaw, Vincent Van Gogh, Leo Tolstoy, Albert Schweitzer, and, of course, India's Mahatma Gandhi.

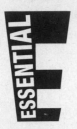

Many contemporary figures, including numerous Hollywood stars, have described themselves as vegetarian, but a spokesman at the Vegetarian Resource Group warns that those who are truly vegetarian are just a fraction of the names usually listed. A celebrity may become a vegetarian for a few years, and then change lifestyles, or may express interest in vegetarian ideals but never make the commitment.

A Growing Movement

Whether health or environmental concerns are propelling the movement forward remains unclear. But statistics show that increasing numbers of Americans and Europeans are switching to a plant-based diet—and many Asians already call themselves vegetarian. As evidence, the growth of vegetarian food items in supermarkets and vegetarian choices in school cafeterias support the notion that for many consumers, this is a movement whose time has come.

Numbers Worldwide

While The International Vegetarian Union (IVU) cannot cite reliable growth figures because the term *vegetarian* has so many different interpretations, its staff does provide a timeline showing the growth of its own membership and affiliations. Still, citing exact figures in various countries is impossible, say the IVU staff, but it has estimated that in the early 1990s, there were these vegetarian totals (the IVU has not done a study since then):

- France: 500,000
- Germany: 700,000

- Netherlands: 700,000
- Poland: 75,000
- Sweden: 60,000
- United Kingdom: 3,500,000

Taking Vegetarian Courses

Considering the growth of the movement in the United States and abroad, it's not surprising that enterprising cooks have set up classes and whole programs to teach how to cook and eat vegetarian. Many of these classes are listed on the web and may be described as holistic or natural health classes.

If you cannot find a course near you, consult your local adult education programs for the names of vegetarian cooking teachers in your community. If that fails, you will be able to sign up for online classes in vegetarianism; this may lead to finding cooking classes or provide tips and recipes for vegetarian cooking.

Dating Services, Travel and Social Groups, and Charities

As with any interest group, vegetarians have set up their own communities to include dating services, travel groups, social and eating clubs, and charities. Once again, the web is a valuable resource for locating any one of these communities. Such groups as Veggiedate.com and Veggieconnection.com give ample links to like-minded people in your area. For travelers, check out the Vegetarian Resource Group, whose website lists several travel services and options specifically for vegetarians. You can also find a series of guidebooks for vegetarian travelers published by *www.vegetarianguides. co.uk*.

Plenty of social and eating clubs are flourishing: check out *http:// vegetarian.meetup.com* or *www.greenpeople.org* to find a group in your community.

As for charities, most are established to raise money to help prevent animal cruelty or to rescue farm animals. In Britain, the Vegetarian Society, with the help of Paul McCartney among others, works to promote vegetarianism and a more compassionate society—and to prevent animal cruelty.

Vegetarian Festivals

During almost every month somewhere in the world, vegetarians gather for celebrations and festivals. For example, during the month of March in Britain, the organization Animal Aid promotes its Veggie Month in support of stopping farm animal slaughter. Starting the first day of spring, thousands of Americans and residents of other countries host "Meatout," grassroots community gatherings that are both fun and informative ways to celebrate a nonmeat diet. For information, check *www.meatout.org*.

October 1 is World Vegetarian Day, and it begins the month-long series of parties and presentations of National Vegetarian Month, also known as Vegetarian Awareness Month. World Vegan Day occurs on November 1, and if you happen to be in Thailand on the island of Phuket during October, you may want to attend the annual Phuket Vegetarian Festival, a colorful if somewhat bizarre series of activities that has its roots in religious practices.

For a comprehensive listing of what's going on and where, check out *www.vegetarianguides.co.uk/calendar/index.shtml*.

Achieving the Switch

If you have decided that vegetarianism makes sense for you and your lifestyle, you may want to start in slowly, learning what you need to eat and trying out the various vegetarian options in your market. Veggies and fruits are one thing, but what about all those different tofu and soy products? How do they fit in?

Plan a week's worth of menus, basing your main dishes on ones you love, but switching out, say, the beef meatballs for vegetarian ones. Or if you are a chili-head, why not create some really appealing meatless chiles, or for that meaty texture, add the taco-seasoned soy ground meat with plenty of beans and salsa for a satisfying entrée.

If cheese is your secret passion and you're a vegan, try any of the shredded or sliced soy cheeses in your favorite recipes. These soy products not only taste and look like meats and dairy cheese, they give nonvegetarians the sense that they can edge into their new diet without feeling deprived of their favorite foods. Even if you get derailed along the way, and keep a few meats and seafood in your menus, you will still feel you've made the great vegetarian leap.

Answering the Nay-Sayers

Once you've started on the path, and friends and family see that you've changed how and what you eat, you may face criticism or teasing. As the Vegetarian Resource Group advises, point out to people that vegetarianism is becoming increasingly popular. Then add that eating a meat-free diet is a personal choice you've made for the following reason or reasons, then list them.

You might also win over others to your way of cooking, living, and eating by preparing delicious vegetarian meals, or at the very least, taking friends and family along when you eat at a vegetarian restaurant. They may be in for a real surprise, especially when they total up the bill and see how reasonable vegetarian food costs can be.

Vegetarian Restaurants

Back in the 1970s, the Moosewood Restaurant in Ithaca, New York, launched a revolutionary restaurant movement by creating and serving outstanding all-vegetarian dishes, inspiring future generations of restaurateurs to follow in their vegetarian footsteps. Since then, not surprisingly, more all-veg restaurants are opening their doors to an influx of new customers—a national Restaurant Association poll from 2001 showed that 1.5 percent of entrées are vegetarian; about eight out of ten restaurants offer vegetarian entrées. Many upscale eateries with white-tablecloth manners have taken up the vegetarian challenge and offer vegetarian options. Even some fast-food outlets are getting in on the act.

While not all cities and towns offer vegetarian restaurant choices, in many communities with an Indian or Chinese population, consumers can readily find South Indian or Chinese Buddhist vegetarian restaurants; these still account for the majority of vegetarian establishments. It's not uncommon for mainstream restaurants to acknowledge that their customer base more frequently requests vegetarian entrées. Note that at least one website offers restaurants a "restaurant starter kit" that tells them what vegetarian consumers look for and how to cook it for them.

Staying Veg

Welcome to the world of vegetarianism meals. You've walked the path successfully, but now you ask yourself, Can I stick to the plan? Of course, but if you feel you need family support, ask for it. Treat yourself to vegetarian cookbooks so that your mealtimes don't become routine and your food boring. And continue to learn about this new lifestyle, perhaps even monitoring any health or energy changes you note. That way, you'll feel positive about the choices you've made and, perhaps, you may even inspire others, too.

CHAPTER 2

Getting the Nutrition You Need

New vegetarians may wonder: What's to eat now that meats are off the table? And newcomers may worry that meals may be bland or monotonous or even very restrictive. But perhaps the most looming concern a vegetarian has is the most important one: Will I get all my nutrients?

What Is a Healthy Vegetarian Diet?

As most experts agree, including the American Dietetic Association, a balanced vegetarian diet does provide all a person's recommended daily nutrients. But there's a catch: not all vegetarians practice the same form of vegetarianism, so no one diet fits all. A new vegetarian's best bet is to become familiar with the key nutrients and where to find them. It may also be worth consulting a registered dietitian or a nutritionist to get the pertinent nutritional information. If you make that choice, be sure to select someone who is well trained and who has had experience in counseling vegetarians and in planning a vegetarian menu.

With knowledge of body chemistry and an understanding of food science, that person can take a medical history, and then question you about what you have been eating, why you are making the dietary change, and what your food likes and dislikes are. He'll know your age and probably also ask about your activity level—if you exercise regularly and are fairly active, your nutritional needs will be higher. Then you two can plan out what your meals should include. That way you can buy, cook, and eat the most wholesome foods.

Whether you consult a dietitian or just map out your own vegetarian plan, you need to know some basics: key nutrients include protein; vitamins D, B12, and A; iron; calcium; and zinc. You will also need a source of omega-3 fatty acids, important for preventing heart disease. Their most abundant natural source comes from fish and fish oils. Unless you are an lacto-ovó vegetarian who uses eggs from hens fed on a diet with omega-3 fatty acids or a pescatarian-vegetarian who eats fish, you need to find another source. Other good sources include flaxseed oil and such vegetable oils as olive oil and canola.

When you are all set, study the Oldways Preservation Trust vegetarian food pyramid (page 16) and write out your shopping list accordingly. You will see that the majority of your food choices and the basics for a sound vegetarian diet will come from the largest food groups: fruits and vegetables, whole grains, and legumes.

If you are a lacto-ovó vegetarian, you should include moderate amounts of dairy products and egg whites, and for added calcium and protein, add in such soy foods as soymilk and soy "meat," analogs, plus be sure to incorporate vegetable oils. The meatlike soy products, such as sausages, bacon, ground beef, and ham, are readily available and add variety to a greens-and-grains-based diet. Best of all, these are lower in fat and calories than their meat counterparts, an important consideration if you have just made the vegetarian switch and are concerned about weight and heart health. At the top of your pyramid are the foods you'll eat the least: whole eggs and sweets.

Since vegans eat no dairy products or eggs, their diets are deficient in and even lack some basics, such as calcium from milk and vitamin B12, a nutrient found exclusively in animal proteins. Vegans may need to add dietary supplements to meet all their nutrient needs and should add fortified foods such as soymilk with added nutrients and fortified breakfast cereals to their daily menu plans.

As you see, you can eat well and live a healthy vegetarian life—but you must learn about what your body needs to stay healthy. Remember: Becoming a vegetarian is not just a matter of abstaining from meat. It requires that vegetarians think about what they are going to eat for the best health, and then to plan accordingly.

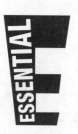

Food pyramids tell the tale: Study the Oldways version on page 16 or click inside the USDA pyramid at *www.mypyramid.gov/pyramid/index .html*, where, if you omit the meats, the USDA pyramid helps you plan your meals. For more information, refer to the USDA's vegetarian tips at *www.mypyramid.gov/tips_resources/vegetarian_diets.html*.

A Vegetarian's Food Plan

As most experts agree, eating the vegetarian way provides you all the necessary nutrients. But as you have learned, there's no single diet and no single source for every nutrient. The key to your success is combining foods from different groups and then getting enough calories to meet your activity and age levels.

To get it right, say the experts at the Oldways Preservation Trust, you'll need several daily servings from the food groups—fruits and vegetables, whole grains, and legumes—at the base of their pyramid. But you should be sure to get moderate servings from all the food levels, and drink enough water each day to stay healthy. Make sure your diet contains the appropriate balance of carbohydrates, fats, and proteins.

The Traditional Healthy Vegetarian Diet Pyramid

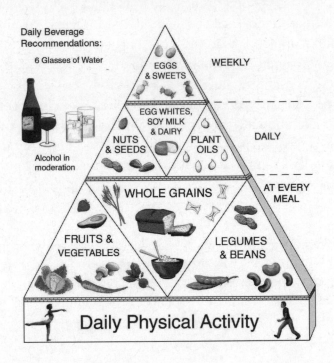

© 2000 Oldways Preservation & Exchange Trust, *www.oldwayspt.org*

The Oldways Preservation Trust staff also stresses that you should avoid processed foods and select, instead, the whole foods that are complete as nature intends them. Processed foods such as grains, sugars, and flours are often stripped of their natural nutrients. Even when vitamins and minerals are added back in later—a process called "enriching," which means that the nutrients lost during refining are added back in to enrich the product—the total effect is never the same.

Take the example of rice: white rice may cook faster and have a more adaptable taste, but by stripping away the outer bran layer, the rice grains loose much of their beneficial fiber and minerals. As proof, one cup of brown rice contains three and a half grams of fiber. One cup of white rice contains less than one gram. Even enriching white rice doesn't make up the difference in the loss of fiber and minerals.

Another confusing term for consumers is *fortifying*, and many of today's foods are fortified with added vitamins and minerals. Fortifying milk with vitamin D is one example; adding folic acid to specific foods is another. *Enriching*, then, means putting back into a refined food nutrients lost during processing; *fortifying* means perhaps adding back lost nutrients, but also adding in others that may not occur naturally in a particular food.

But processing or refining plant foods can also destroy the complex plant chemicals known as phytonutrients, or phytochemicals. Many of these naturally occurring chemicals have health-supporting benefits and have been used for centuries for their antioxidant, anti-inflammatory, and anti-carcinogenic properties. Considering that salicin extracted from the white willow tree has been a long-term painkiller and the basis for today's aspirin, it's easy to understand why unprocessed fruits and vegetables can be your body's best friends.

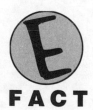

According to the USDA, phytonutrients may act as antioxidants, cause cancer cells to die, repair DNA damaged from smoking, and improve the body's immune response.

Daily Needs and Food Sources

According to Katherine Tallmadge, a spokesperson for the American Dietetic Association and a practicing nutritionist, the daily diet program following on the next page, based on the ADA guidelines, should guide vegetarians to eat right.

Milk and Milk Alternatives Group: Six to Eight Servings Daily

- ½ cup milk, yogurt, or fortified soymilk
- ¾ ounce natural cheese
- ½ to 1 cup cottage cheese
- ¼ cup calcium-set tofu
- 1 cup cooked dry beans, such as soy, cannellini, pinto, navy, great northern, kidney, and black beans
- ¼ cup shelled almonds
- 3 tablespoons sesame tahini or almond butter
- 1 cup cooked or 2 cups raw bok choy, Chinese cabbage, broccoli, collards, kale, or okra
- 1 tablespoon blackstrap molasses
- 5 figs

Dry Beans, Nuts, Seeds, Eggs, and Meat Substitutes Group: Two to Three Servings Daily

- 1 cup cooked dry beans, lentils, or peas
- 2 cups soymilk
- ½ cup tofu or tempeh
- 2 ounces vegetarian "meats" or soy cheese
- 2 eggs or 4 egg whites
- ¼ cup nuts or seeds
- 3 tablespoons nut or seed butters

Fruit Group: Two to Four Servings Daily

- ¾ cup juice
- ¼ cup dried fruit
- ½ cup chopped raw fruit
- ½ cup canned fruit
- 1 medium-size piece of fruit such as banana, apple, or orange

Vegetable Group: Three to Five Servings Daily

- ½ cup cooked or chopped raw vegetables
- 1 cup raw, leafy vegetables
- ¾ cup vegetable juice

Bread, Cereal, Rice, and Pasta Group: Six to Eleven Servings Daily
- 1 slice (1 ounce) bread
- ½ small bagel, bun or English muffin (or 1 ounce)
- 1 ounce ready-to-eat cereal
- 2 tablespoons wheat germ
- ½ cup cooked (1 ounce dry) grains, cereal, rice, or pasta

Fats, Oils, Sweets: Use Sparingly
- Candy, butter, dairy fats, solid margarine (high in trans fats)

Do Raw Foods Count?

Some vegetarians follow a raw-foods diet, but they should take special care with the fruits and vegetables they eat. According to the Centers for Disease Control (CDC), raw animal foods—even eggs and raw milk—may contain pathogens. But CDC scientists point out that any raw food exposed to a contaminated food source can contain pathogens.

Likewise, pathogens can readily contaminate raw fruits and vegetables, particularly if these were processed in unsanitary conditions, were fertilized with contaminated manure, or were washed for packing in unclean water. Even unpasteurized fruit juices may be unsafe if made from contaminated fresh fruits. Washing whole fresh produce at home may diminish but not totally eliminate any pathogens. See Chapter 4 for how to keep your foods safe.

Going Organic?

Going green and *eating sustainable foods* are buzzwords for the twenty-first century. But these terms underscore what consumers need to know about their food supply. The underlying message is that consumers should buy as much locally grown food as available; by doing that you support local agriculture, cut down on transportation costs and fuel bills, and eat produce that is both seasonal and fresh.

As for eating organic foods, it's an industry hot-button subject, because not everyone agrees that foods grown without pesticides and synthetic fertilizers are any healthier than those grown according to more conventional methods. But at least some food and plant scientists are making the case that organic, or natural, farming gives foods some disease-fighting abilities.

For example, plants contain a micronutrient known as flavonoids that, according to the scientists at the Linus Pauling Institute at Oregon State University, may benefit people by protecting against heart disease and certain cancers. Flavonoids may also help boost the immune system and work as an antioxidant. Some sources claim that organically raised plant foods are better able to produce flavonoids; when sprayed with chemicals, plants lose some of that ability. In addition, plants not sprayed with pesticides don't carry any harmful residue that humans may consume.

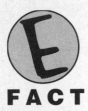

According to a May 2008 article on the Inter Press Service, even China and its farmers are joining the organics boom, not only to satisfy foreign demand, but also to feed Chinese city dwellers, who prefer crops grown on chemical-free lands.

Getting Down to Basics: Protein

What are proteins? Proteins are made up of amino acids, which are a protein's building blocks. Twenty different amino acids combine to form all the proteins the body needs. Some of these amino acids can't be made by your body, so you have to get them from a food source: these are known as essential amino acids. Complete proteins such as milk, eggs, cheese, and meat sources provide these essential amino acids. An incomplete protein contains only small amounts of one or several amino acids.

What Proteins Do

Proteins are the body's main building blocks, the vital nutrients that fuel the body's ability to grow and maintain itself in good health and to help ward off infections. In fact, every cell in your body, including your skin, hair, and nails, contains proteins. Eating enough protein can also help you keep fit and trim and even lose a few unwanted pounds. Next to water, protein accounts for the largest component in your body. But your body's proteins are in constant flux, always being renewed and replaced as your cells grow and repair themselves.

Protein Sources

Animal-based diets obviously provide plenty of protein, but eating a varied plant-based diet can, too. Dairy foods such as milk, cheese, and yogurt are excellent protein sources. Such nondairy sources as eggs, beans, and soy products, even fruits and seeds, contain enough proteins to round out the typical vegetarian diet.

How much protein do people need? According to the CDC, the recommended daily allowance (RDA) for protein for adult women is forty-six grams a day; for adult men, fifty-six grams a day. A well-planned and varied vegetarian diet for any age group will contain enough daily proteins. The USDA's MyPyramid shows how vegetarians can get enough proteins if their diet includes beans; nuts; nut butters; peas; soy products; and, for lacto-ovó vegetarians, eggs.

Complementary Proteins

Because not all proteins are alike, some experts say that you need to build complete proteins by combining amino acids or protein sources so that you eat enough complete proteins. Complementary proteins are two or more incomplete protein sources that together provide adequate amounts of all the essential amino acids. Some experts insist that combining protein sources—say, combining rice with beans with their differing types of amino acids—provides all the essential amino acids.

Others disagree, saying that the myth of complementary proteins is just that, a myth. Eating a varied plant diet with ample calories assures vegetarians they are getting complete proteins. Who has the final say? For your needs, talk to a nutritionist.

The Body's Spark Plugs: Vitamins and Minerals

While all vitamins and minerals play an important role in how well your body functions, vegetarians should pay special attention to these: iron, calcium, vitamin B12, and zinc.

Iron

Plenty has been written about how the body needs iron for red blood cells and carrying oxygen throughout the body. Plenty has also been written about how iron deficiency leads to anemia, a condition characterized by fatigue, insomnia, and weakness, and one that commonly occurs in women and children. Vegetarians can get plenty of iron by including spinach, kidney beans, lentils, blackstrap molasses, and whole wheat baked goods. If you feel you are iron deficient, consult a nutritionist.

Calcium

As informed consumers know, calcium is the key mineral needed for forming and maintaining strong bones and teeth, but it also helps it with other body functions. To get enough calcium, vegetarians should eat calcium-fortified foods, soy products, and plenty of leafy greens, and, of course, dairy products.

Vitamin B12

Your body may need only small amounts of vitamin B12, but it is essential for the proper growth of red blood cells and for the health of some nerve tissues. Signs of a B12 deficiency include numbness and tingling in hands and legs, weakness, disorientation, and depression, among others. Because vitamin B12 occurs in animal proteins, lacto-ovó vegetarians should get plenty in their daily diet by eating eggs and dairy products. Vegans, however, need to find an alternate source, such as flaxseed oil or nutritional yeast.

Zinc

You've heard about taking a zinc supplement if you begin to feel sick? That's because the mineral zinc helps bolster the immune system. But as the Office of Dietary Supplements at the National Institutes of Health in Bethesda, Maryland, points out, zinc also helps heal wounds and helps sustain the senses of smell and taste. Zinc occurs naturally in red meat and poultry, in some seafood, and in beans, nuts, whole grains, and dairy products.

Do You Need Dietary Supplements?

Should you or shouldn't you? That's the question that has caused plenty of controversy between the medical profession and the health-food supporters, with everyone taking up one side or the other. According to Congress in the Dietary Supplement Health and Education Act, which became law in 1994, a dietary supplement is one that contains one or more dietary ingredients, including vitamins, minerals, and/or amino acids, plus other possible ingredients, and is intended to add nutrients to a diet that could be deficient.

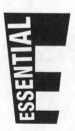

Since vegetarians may feel their diet lacks certain nutrients, they may reach for the vitamin or mineral pill to fill in the gaps. But the wise person should seek medical or health care advice before taking any supplements. For further information, check out the Office of Dietary Supplements website at *www.ods.od.nih.gov.*

Many manufacturers make claims for their supplement products; some claims may seem outlandish, and others may even be fraudulent. For your own protection and that of your loved ones, you should be the wary consumer: get the facts and make some educated choices—particularly essential for the vegetarian population.

According to the FDA, supplements should not be used to replace a balanced diet. Consumers should also be aware that those with particular health problems and who are taking supplements may face some unintended results: the supplements may interact with prescription or over-the-counter drugs or for the presurgical patient, a supplement may cause dangerous interactions during surgery.

Filling Up on Fiber

You've probably heard it all before, and even seen all the television commercials telling you how to get enough fiber each day—eat this cereal, take that pill. You may end up wondering whether you can possibly eat what you need for your daily requirements. The answer is "yes." You don't need to take anything extra, because you get plenty of fiber in your diet by following a vegetarian eating plan.

What Is Fiber?

A type of carbohydrate, fiber is found in all plant foods, including whole grains and legumes, and is an indigestible carbohydrate. It occurs in two forms: insoluble fiber, which helps prevent constipation; and soluble fiber, which helps lower blood cholesterol levels. Women should eat about twenty grams of fiber each day; men, thirty-plus grams. Most Americans eat far less fiber each day than they should. If you are on a fiber-poor diet, add fiber slowly, and always drink plenty of water each day.

What Does Dietary Fiber Do?

Fiber plays several important roles in your health by adding the roughage, or bulk, that keeps your digestive tract working smoothly. Because your body cannot absorb or digest it, fiber also slows down the digestive process so that glucose gets absorbed more slowly, and that helps keep blood sugar levels stable and reduces the risks of obesity and certain cancers.

How to Slip Fiber into Your Diet

At the market, select fiber-rich foods; all plants contain fiber, but some, such as beans, potatoes, and apples, are richer sources than others. Then when possible, eat your fruits and vegetables unpeeled or whole. For example, if you give up your morning orange juice and eat the orange instead, you get two and a half grams of fiber instead of less than one gram from the juice. And eat the whole baked potato, skin and all.

Add bulk each day by choosing a big salad for lunch, and garnishing it with beans and maybe some cooked grains. For dinner, load up on two servings of vegetables, or fix a big vegetable stir-fry garnished with tofu and seasoned with your choice of Asian condiments.

When you buy sandwich breads, look for the whole-grain varieties and leave the white breads behind. Remember that the fiber has been processed out of white flours; one exception is the product known as "white whole wheat flour," which has good baking qualities suitable for cakes and pastries.

CHAPTER 3

Shopping Vegetarian

Perhaps the best part of any foodie's life is thinking about the many ingredient choices in the marketplace. This is especially true if you are one of those people who have changed—gradually or suddenly—from a meat-based diet to a vegetarian way of cooking and eating. You'll love how many delicious vegetarian ingredients you can cook up—plus you can find vegetarian-friendly cosmetics, household products, and even vegetarian pet food.

Setting Up the Vegetarian Kitchen

Regardless of where your passions lie, eating daily is a must, and cooking—unless you are on a raw food or take-out diet—is all part of the plan. So your best bet is to look at the process with a positive eye and learn, if you don't already know, how to make your kitchen become your best friend.

For new vegetarians, there's plenty to learn—actually, a whole new vocabulary of shopping, cooking, and eating. Such words or terms as "tempeh" and "soy meat alternatives" and even "natural sweeteners" may be totally unfamiliar. If that's the case, you should educate yourself—learn the lingo and get comfortable with this vast world of vegetarian staples you are embracing.

Regardless of how long you've been a vegetarian, the vegetarian kitchen may still seem hard to decode. If so, read through some vegetarian and vegan cookbooks. Then check what's available on the many websites. For example, one of the classiest places to start learning about good vegetarian cooking is the Food Network at *www.foodnetwork.com/food.* Its chefs and recipe collections are considered some of the best in the marketplace, and selecting recipes there assures you of some decidedly upscale eating.

You can also find cooking inspiration at the Vegetarian Resource Group, *www.vrg.org*; the International Vegetarian Union, *www.ivu.org/recipes*; and for all-vegan fare, *www.vegweb.com.*

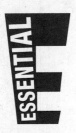

Plenty of helpful vegetarian cookbooks, like Deborah Madison's *Vegetarian Suppers* and her classics *The Greens Cookbook* and *Vegetarian Cooking for Everyone*, and all the cookbooks in the Moosewood Restaurant series, should give you ample ideas to set out on a full-fledged vegetarian-cooking bonanza.

Shopping Veg

Urban dwellers may be particularly fortunate, for chances are that organic food markets, ethnic grocers, international specialty stores, and well-stocked supermarkets are within easy reach. For them, the choices are infinite, and the shopping pleasures, many.

As you will discover, most supermarkets now carry enough vegetarian goods so that you don't need to chase them down at health food stores or order hard-to-find items over the web. Just about anything you could possibly want for your pantry is right at hand.

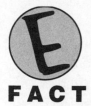

FACT

Shopping veg means that you can buy not only vegetarian food ingredients but also assorted other veg products. Want to feed Fido a vegetarian diet? If so, go to a pet store or buy a product online. You can even cook up your own, but before you change Fido's diet, check with your vet. Dogs (and cats) are naturally carnivores, though dogs can subsist on a diet for omnivores. See page 37.

Where to Start

Make friends with your kitchen. As with any kitchen setting, the vegetarian kitchen—even if you are the only one in the household on a plant-based diet—needs some adjusting. For example, your pantry may need a makeover that's more veg-friendly.

This doesn't mean that you have to discard what other family members choose to eat. If your children, husband, or significant other still enjoy their chicken cutlets, for example, keep them in the freezer, but make room for what's important to you.

Basic Pantry Items

This is really about going back to the basics. Think about those possible meals when you will be too tired or too rushed to slow-cook a grains-based meal. That's when you'll miss out on some good eating, especially if you don't have your pantry stocked with such basics as canned beans, already made vegetable broth and soups, and plenty of dried herbs. Such staples are handy when you run out of time and energy but still want a tasty meal.

You can also stock up on aseptically packaged tofu and soymilk, sealed packets of seaweed to top your miso soup, handy prepacked soup mixes, energy bars, and even a good supply of ready-to-eat nuts and seeds. Some markets also sell precooked and vacuum-packed brown and wild rice and noodles. So look at your cupboards, rethink your eating plans, then make your pantry and fridge fit into your lifestyle.

Don't forget about filling your freezer with ready-made vegetarian entrées and "burgers." Most major brands produce some vegetarian products, so scout out the freezer cases.

Other Vegetarian Staples

Like to experiment with ethnic dishes, but don't have time to race around town regularly? Take several hours of your free time some weekend, and stock up on loads of basics. At an Indian grocery, you'll find lentils of every color, to say nothing of a slew of exotic spices. Hispanic markets are good sources for dried beans of many different varieties, and often these come in economy-size bags for budget-conscious shoppers.

Love Asian noodles? Asian markets will seem like a treasure chest, for you can pick up dried noodles from China, Vietnam, Japan, and Thailand in one stop. You may even find seasoning staples such as fresh lemongrass, assorted makes of canned coconut milk, and seasoning pastes and sauces to suit every palate. If you plan to cook within a few days after shopping, bring home some of the fresh noodle varieties and add to your basket some of the assorted fresh tofu products.

Sugars Versus Natural Sweeteners

Many vegetarians spurn granulated sugars, as some manufacturers produce it by filtering raw cane sugars through charred animal bones. It's impossible for consumers to know how the sugar is produced, so vegetarians should turn to other natural sweeteners. Vegans won't sweeten foods with honey because it is the product of living creatures, and eating honey is considered exploiting bees.

Whether or not you omit these sweeteners from your pantry doesn't mean you can't add a dash of something sweet to your pan. Agave nectar, date sugar, maple syrup, and stevia are perfectly sweet and perfectly acceptable; however, except for pure maple syrup, the other products may be more difficult to find. For more information on sweeteners, see Chapter 15.

Oils, Fats, and Nonstick Cooking Sprays

With all the fuss about trans fats, hydrogenated fats, and heart health, picking out what's healthiest is important. Every diet should include some oils, and you should keep quality olive oils—preferably extra virgin oils for heightening flavors, though not really for cooking—on hand. But the trick is to keep fat intake down, even if your fat source is a so-called healthy oil.

You should also select a good-quality vegetable oil, such as peanut or canola oil, for your sautéing and stir-frying. If you are a vegan, you will exclude butter, but you should select a good nonhydrogenated margarine instead, one that does not contain the animal product whey. And if you really are looking to trim fats, keep a container on hand of nonstick cooking spray: this could become indispensable for any quick pan-frying you do.

Specialty oils useful for adding a flavor profile include toasted sesame oil, hazelnut oil, and walnut oil. Some vegetarian cooks replace fat in baking with such ingredients as applesauce and mashed bananas.

Flours

The next time you browse the baking aisle, check out the many types of flours on sale: the options may seem bewildering—from pastry flours, to self-rising flours, to cake flours, to the general all-purpose types. So here's your chance to know ahead what is in the bag. For general all-purpose baking, the all-purpose white flours are fine, but look for a brand that at least is unbleached, and better yet, also contains flour from organic wheat or other grains.

Whole wheat flours are fine for sturdier baked goods, but they don't produce as fine a crumb and are not really suitable for delicate pastries. Yet because these flours still contain the whole bran and wheat germ, they contain more nutrients. Relatively new to the marketplace are the white whole wheat flours, which contain all the nutrients and fiber of whole wheat flours but bake up like pastry flours. Several manufacturers retail this product made from organically grown wheats, a double benefit for the consumer. For more about flours, see Chapter 15.

Food Labeling

It's become most people's habit to read food labels, especially to figure out the calorie counts, fat grams, and amounts of added sugars—such as sucrose, fructose, or glucose—and the amounts of sodium. Sodium levels can be particularly high with canned beans, and even if you like using the liquid packed with the beans, you'd be better off draining and rinsing the beans—and getting rid of excess sodium—before you use them.

As you look for whole-grain items, be sure that the word "whole-grain" comes first or second on the ingredients list; otherwise you may be getting a product that is not as wholesome as you want.

If you do stock up on canned goods, you should check that the products you buy are as free of added chemicals and preservatives as possible. You'll also want to wise up on the number of servings and the calorie counts per serving—nutrition labels tell you what you find in one serving only—do not make the mistake that the figures refer to the entire contents.

Raw Vegetables and Fruits Count

Thanks to the efforts of the U.S. Food and Drug Administration (FDA), retailers are more often providing shoppers with some basic nutritional information for the twenty most popular varieties of fruits and vegetables—including such items as peaches, pears, plums, cucumbers, cauliflower, and broccoli—in the produce bins. The information includes the name of the item, a suggested serving size, and the calories per serving. The labeling is voluntary, but many retailers are complying with the FDA's request.

The Whys of Vegetarian and Vegan Labeling

When shopping, you must also learn to check the fine print: some manufacturers may disguise the fact that their product contains some animal product or products. Such ingredients as casein, rennet, gelatin, and glycerides all come from animals.

As the Vegetarian Resource Group points out, retailers now often package their vegetarian products with a vegetarian or vegan symbol. Finding such a symbol or all-veg food label should reassure you that what you are buying is animal-product free, but there are no government agencies that enforce this kind of labeling.

When Labels Say "Organic"

Even though no federal regulations control the labeling of vegetarian and vegan foods, government-approved certifiers do oversee the labeling of organic foods; if the label reads "organic," then you can be sure it has been produced according to the strict laws supervising foods grown and labeled organic. That means what you are buying must contain 95 to 100 percent organic ingredients, and that the ingredients are grown without pesticides or other harmful chemicals added.

Buying fresh organically raised fruits and vegetables, however, does not mean you don't have to wash your produce at home before using it. While your fruits and vegetables may not have been sprayed with pesticides, they may have been exposed to sprays and other chemicals just from the effects of natural weather conditions.

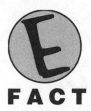

FACT

The USDA has established the National Organic Program, which requires that agricultural products labeled as "100 percent" organic must be just that, 100 percent organic, excluding water and salt. To find out more about this and all other food labeling, go to *http://fnic.nal.usda.gov/nal_display/index.php?info_center=4&tax_level=1.*

Alternative Markets

Many consumers are looking elsewhere, outside of the big-box supermarkets, for their basic ingredients. Today's consumer push for a greener environment and safer food production and food sources have brought a whole new dimension to food shopping and to cooking.

A couple of labels the savvy consumer takes seriously these days are "sustainable" and "local." Buying produce that is grown in the rural farming areas near where you live—therefore, native to the climate and soil in your region—is a way of getting both local *and* sustainable foods.

Sustainable foods are grown in ways that don't harm the environment and that help save our natural resources. And a locally grown product means that you aren't paying for the shipping costs levied on merchants for importing foods from hundreds or thousands of miles away.

Health Food and Natural Foods Stores and Cooperatives

In the mid-to-late twentieth century, the few resources for buying either vegetarian or wholesome whole foods were limited to health food or natural foods stores. Appealing to a small segment of the population, these stores were, however, reliable sources for grains, supplements, and hard-to-find food supplies such as brewer's yeast and blackstrap molasses.

Customer- or staff-owned food co-ops have been consistent sources for stocking and selling natural foods and vegetarian products as well as for providing educational materials and, often, cooking classes and recipes. Both still play a valuable role in providing shoppers with nourishing choices. But today's concerned consumer has spurred the growth of mainstream markets that now stock what were once considered "fringe" items.

CSAs

Community-supported agriculture, or CSAs, provide a way for the consumer to buy into, or subscribe to, a farmer's weekly production of vegetables, fruits, eggs, and other farm goods. This benefits both the farmer, who is assured of selling what he grows, and the consumer, who gets weekly deliveries of farm-fresh goods. Most areas of the country have nearby farmers who participate in a CSA. To check out what's available near you, log onto *www.localharvest.org/csa*.

Farmers' Markets

Farm stands are as American as apple pie, but they have their counterpart in large weekly farmers' markets in most cities abroad. Tourists who want to understand a country's culture always make the city marketplace their first stop.

Americans got out of the habit of buying from their local farmers and local farm stands once supermarkets arrived and made one-stop shopping so convenient. But the resurgence of farmers' markets portends a different consumer attitude about buying fresh and buying local.

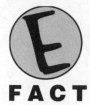

FACT

According to the USDA, as of 2008 more than 4,600 farmers' markets operated nationwide, and the demand for them continues to grow. For more information, check out *www.ams.usda.gov/farmersmarkets*.

Even in the nation's capital, shopping at the farmers' markets operated by the group FRESHfarm Markets has become something of a weekly social event, particularly at the Dupont Circle location on Sundays. For many, shopping there is as important as attending a congressman's dinner party. Unless you are actually a farmer, where else can you feel a part of how and where your food grows? What better way to stay connected to the land than by striking up a relationship with the person who works it and grows what you eat? For more information, check out *http://apps.ams.usda.gov/Farmers Markets*, or *www.localharvest.org/farmers-markets*, or call your local agricultural extension service.

Become an Activist

If joining groups and supporting causes are new to you, this is as good a time as any to volunteer for one of the many environmental groups that lobby Congress or try to educate the dining public about the values of farmland and food production. These causes complement many aspects of vegetarianism—sometimes referred to as "environmental vegetarianism"—when they touch on the need to preserve our environment, to reduce the use of fossil fuels, and to keep our food sources safe from pollution.

Several groups working actively to educate people about the environment, about supporting sustainable agriculture, and about preserving our food culture include Slow Food USA at *www.slowfoodusa.org*; Sierra Club at *www.sierraclub.org*; The Nature Conservancy at *www.nature.org*; the Orion Grassroots Network at *www.orionsociety.org*; and American Farmland Trust at *www.farmland.org*. To locate which group is nearest you, use the Internet and join to support the health of our planet and our farmlands.

Household Supplies, Cosmetics, and Toiletries

What else is going green? If you think that green living pertains only to foods, conserving gasoline and electricity, and some household detergents, you might be very surprised to find that enterprising manufacturers have gone beyond the conventional consumer products to supply the marketplace with everything environmentally sound—and usually vegetarian friendly—from insect repellants to lipsticks to non-GMO seeds. Even baby clothes made from natural organic cottons are available, as are picnic supplies, clothing, and furniture polish, all of which are kind to the environment and are humanely manufactured.

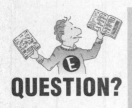

QUESTION?

What is a GMO?
A GMO is a genetically modified organism, which means for plants that their genetic makeup, or DNA, has been modified with genetic engineering techniques. While that may increase crop yield and some disease resistance, it also alters nature and has an unknown impact on agriculture and human health. See Chapter 10 to learn about non-GMO soy products.

The British and Australians seem savvier than Americans when it comes to shopping for vegetarian/vegan/environmentally free goods. Several groups such as England's The Vegetarian Society at *www.vegsoc.org* and Australia's the Vegetarian Network Victoria at *www.vnv.org.au* offer consumers leads to finding the best all-veg products. But Americans are catching up: Look for goods and sources at:

- The Vegan Connection at *www.veganconnection.com/info.html*
- The Vegetarian Site at *www.thevegetariansite.com*
- Vegetarians in Paradise at *www.vegparadise.com/linkswe.html*
- Greenpeople at *www.greenpeople.org*

Reading Labels

Labels on food products give you needed information about what you are buying. But the same can be said of labels on nonfood products, such as household supplies, cosmetics, and even toiletries. Look for goods that are labeled saying that they are produced without any animal by-products, are safe for the environment, and that may state "cruelty free." If you are not sure what to look for, check out the Vegetarian Resource Group at *www.vrg.org*.

Vegetarian Pet Supplies

What can companion animals eat? You might think twice about feeding Fido or Tabby some brands of commercial pet foods, especially when you understand what those labels mean: meat by-products could be any part of an animal, from intestines to hooves and processed from any animal source—dead, diseased, or even an animal disabled before slaughter.

Few experts seem to agree on whether a vegetarian diet is really suitable for dogs and cats. Before you make the choice for your animal, discuss the options with your vet, and also check online at *www.aspca.org/aspcablog/2007/06/nutrition-q-vegetarian-diets-for-dogs.html*.

Vegetarian Dogs

Dogs are carnivorous, right? Or, at least, omnivorous. But according to the results of one study solicited through People for the Ethical Treatment of Animals (PETA) of dogs eating a no-meat/no-meat-product diet, the results were gratifying: the dogs studied seemed to thrive. But if you are thinking of switching Fido to a vegetarian diet, you should ask your vet's advice first, then buy commercially prepared vegetarian dog food products that are balanced for all the nutrients dogs require. Make sure that the product says that it is certified by the Association of American Feed Control Officials (AAFCO). This means the food meets the standards for canine nutrition.

If you have put your dog on a vegetarian diet, you will know he is not doing well if he has diarrhea, vomiting, weight or energy loss, or other chronic health conditions with no other obvious reasons. If the dog's food is all-vegan, you might consider adding such protein sources as yogurt or eggs to the diet. For more information, check out *www.vegetarian-central.com* or *www.vegetariandogs.com*.

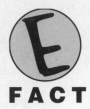

FACT

Whether or not you put your pet on a vegetarian diet, you can at least outfit your dog or cat with all-natural, environmentally friendly shampoos, flea therapy, dog treats and toys, and training aids. Check out *www .botanicaldog.com* or *www.onlynaturalpet.com*.

Vegetarian Cats

Unlike dogs, cats are carnivores and require certain elements not found in an all-plant diet, including taurine (an amino acid) and arachidonic acid (an essential fatty acid), so not everyone agrees that an all-vegetarian diet is cat-safe. If you are considering putting your cat on such a diet, consult your veterinarian first. For more information about vegetarian cats, go to *www .vegsoc.org/info/catfood.html* or *www.vegetariancats.com*.

CHAPTER 4

Cooking Vegetarian

Maybe you are an old hand at tackling kitchen tasks. Or maybe it's day one of your new vegetarian life. And if you have spent more time warming meals up in the microwave than cooking them from scratch, you may need to hone your cooking skills. Either way, join in the fun! Get cooking . . . and eating!

Brushing Up on the Basics

If you are starting from scratch, get out your notepad and start with your lists. Figuring out the basics is also a good time to learn. Besides a refresher course on the basics, such as steaming, boiling, and pan-frying, you might want to tackle more complicated cooking tasks: stir-frying, roasting, and poaching may be new to your repertoire. Besides, you might be surprised to learn that you can grill and sauté vegetarian ingredients, cooking methods often associated with typical meat-based dishes.

You've learned about reading labels so you won't accidentally pick up any product that contains meat or meat by-products. You've also read about reading labels for nutritional information. But there's much more to think about when you stroll through your produce section or visit the local farmers' markets. For one, you want to pick out the freshest fruit or veggie you can find, avoiding those with obvious bruises or rotten spots. And that's just the beginning. Once you get your foods home, you'll need to know how to store and handle them to avoid contamination or spoilage.

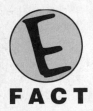

FACT

Be sure your kitchen is outfitted with quality knives—nothing worse than dealing with dull blades that hack your food apart rather than giving it a good, clean slice. A selection of good cookware offers you the chance to experiment and turn out properly cooked meals.

Take stock of your equipment. If you've been working with hand-me-downs or inexpensive discount products, invest in your cooking by buying a good cast iron skillet, a steamer or steamer basket, a rice cooker, saucepans in several sizes, a portable or upright electric mixer, a blender and/or food processor, and even a wok.

Stocking the Staples

Sensible cooks of every persuasion stock their cupboards—and refrigerator and freezer—with some handy items, not only for use in emergency situations, but also for everyday cooking. Some examples include:

Dry Goods
- Baking powder, baking soda, and cornstarch
- Rice, including long-grain white rice, such as jasmine or basmati, and brown rice
- Legumes, such as canned and dried beans, split peas, and lentils
- Whole grains, including cracked wheat, cornmeal, and quinoa
- Flours
- Sweeteners
- Pastas, both dried and fresh
- Hot and cold cereals

Condiments and Seasonings
- Soy sauce; low-sodium soy sauce is a healthful choice
- Vinegars, such as balsamic, white, and herbed
- Extracts, including vanilla, lemon, and almond extracts
- Herbs such as dried oregano, dried thyme, ground turmeric, and ground cumin
- Spices such as ground cinnamon and cinnamon sticks, ground nutmeg, ground cloves, and ground ginger
- Ketchup, mustard, and mayonnaise
- Pickles and relishes
- Beverages, including tea leaves, coffee beans, and fruit juices. Also keep handy soymilks and whole milks in steri-packed cartons.
- Oils, including olive oil and canola oil

For the Refrigerator
Although some items are perishable, these are handy in a pinch:

- Nut butters
- Tofu of varying textures
- Tempeh
- Dairy foods, such as cheese and yogurt

For the Freezer
What you store away for future use can save you cooking headaches on those days when you have no free time for cooking:

- Frozen cooked-ahead meals
- Boxes of frozen vegetables
- Premade pie crusts
- Commercial vegetarian breakfast and dinner entrées and pasta dishes

Cookware and Appliances

Stocking up on cookware and kitchen appliances can be costly, so study what's on the market and make your selections wisely. At the very least, you'll need a skillet, preferably a cast iron one that you can season to make nonstick—many top chefs insist on using cast iron cookware.

Select saucepans of varying sizes and purchase at least one large stockpot for cooking pastas and soups and steaming bulky vegetables, such as artichokes. Select several wooden cooking spoons, a spatula, a roasting pan and cake pans, a colander, a griddle, a vegetable steamer, and measuring cups and spoons. Other basics include a sturdy plastic cutting board or two; a flat or box cheese grater, and possibly a microplane for zesting citrus fruits and grating fresh nutmeg.

As for appliances, you may want a rice cooker—these come in many different sizes and price ranges, but small, reliable, and inexpensive models are readily available. A blender and/or a food processor is a must, as is an upright or hand-held set of electric beaters. A wok is handy for your Asian meals, and some cooks rely on an electric wok, because top models heat up quickly and get hot enough for fast stir-frying—if you choose one, pick out a wok that has a lid and a nonstick cooking surface. Many cooks invest in a slow cooker; these labor- and time-saving appliances take the stress out of mealtimes because you can come home to table-ready meals without stirring the pot once.

Cutlery

As any professional chef knows, good knives are a major investment, and while a vegetarian home cook may not need a meat chopper or a boning or fish knife, you will need high-quality carbon steel knives; these sharpen more easily and stay sharper longer than others. Consider buying a paring knife, a utility knife with an eight- to ten-inch blade (or both), a serrated knife for slicing breads and pastries, and a long slicing knife.

Avoid buying a set of knives that come packaged together, because you may end up with tools you probably can't use. And don't invest in knives that supposedly never need sharpening, because the cutting edges eventually become dull. And to keep your knives razor sharp, you'll need a good knife sharpener. Ask your knife vendor or cookware store staff for the best sharpener in your price range.

Food Safety

Fresh fruits and vegetables should make up a substantial portion of your diet: checking out the Oldways Food Pyramid and the USDA's MyPyramid shows that a healthful diet consists of plentiful servings of fresh vegetables and fruits each day—and you have an abundant choice at most markets.

But even if the produce manager stocks clean shelves, the danger of contamination still lurks—just remember the 2006 E. coli bacteria scare with fresh spinach. No matter how carefully the farmer, the middlemen, and the supermarket staff handle produce, it's possible that the fertilizer and/or the water supply could be contaminated. But consumers can take many steps to protect their food and their health. The FDA advises consumers to select fresh-looking, nonbruised items and to buy cut-up fruits or vegetables that are carefully packaged and chilled or stored on shaved ice.

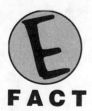
FACT

For a complete rundown on how to select and buy the best produce, check out *www.cfsan.fda.gov/~dms/prodsafe.html#buying*. Another government source of good information: *www.health.gov/dietaryguidelines/ dga2005/document/html/chapter10.htm*.

Safe Food Storage

Back at home, take charge of how your food is stored until you are ready to cook. First, be sure your refrigerator is set to 40°F or lower and that your freezer is set at 0°F or lower. Then refrigerate perishables promptly, especially in summertime heat. Label and date any foods you plan to freeze. Frozen foods have a longer storage life, though their flavor and quality may deteriorate, and freezing does not kill any bacteria present.

High-acid canned goods like citrus fruits have a twelve- to eighteen-month shelf life; low-acid goods like beans can keep safely for at least two years. But check the goods often; you don't know how long these were stocked on your supermarket's shelves. When you see that a can is bulging or leaking, discard it at once.

Grains and legumes are subject to aging, and their natural oils may turn rancid or get bugs, no matter how well you've packaged and stored them. Whenever possible store these in the refrigerator for safest keeping.

If a power outage occurs, keep your freezer door tightly closed; the foods should stay safe for up to two days, provided your freezer has been set to 0°F. Fruits—such as whole blueberries or cranberries—that thaw slightly and then are refrozen may develop ice crystals or become mushy when totally thawed. You may want to discard them or use them in a fruit dessert or drink. According to the FDA, you may refreeze a food before cooking it if it has thawed in the refrigerator.

Handling Precooked Foods or Leftovers

If you have planned ahead and cooked several meals for future use, you can keep them safe by cooling the food slightly, then immediately refrigerating the food in tightly sealed containers. Or you can freeze them in portioned sizes in tightly sealed containers.

If you have leftovers you want to save, pack them up immediately; you must discard any perishables left out at room temperature longer than two hours, or for longer than one hour in summer heat. Plan to use up any leftovers within a few days.

Prep Tips

Learning to rinse, clean, and cut up foods safely are basic kitchen-safety measures. Because you can't really see or taste harmful bacteria, the USDA has launched a public campaign to teach consumers how to handle foods to prevent food-borne illnesses. To do so, the USDA has established an enterprise called The Partnership for Food Safety Education at *www.fightbac.org*. The Partnership's basic food-handling guidelines are:

- **Clean:** Wash hands and surfaces often.
- **Separate:** Don't cross contaminate.
- **Cook:** Cook to proper temperatures.
- **Chill:** Refrigerate promptly.

These rules must seem like common sense, but think about it: do you wash your hands for twenty seconds in warm, sudsy water before and after handling foods, after petting the dog, or after touching or handling trash or other dirty surfaces? Do you wear disposable gloves if your hands have any skin infection or cuts?

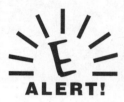

The most important rule for cooking and eating safely: Keep hot foods hot and cold foods cold.

You must take the same precautions with any surfaces, such as a cutting board or knife blade, that come in contact with your food. For example, you should wash cutting boards with soapy water after each use, run them through the dishwasher at day's end, and safely sanitize them with a solution of one teaspoon bleach to one quart water.

Washing Produce Before Use

You are just back from the market with a bagful of goodies. The apples look clean, and you see only a few grains of dirt on the lettuce. Into the fridge right away? No. All produce needs a rinse-off before use; you can't be sure how it's grown or who has handled it before you bring it home. Besides, most produce—especially leafy greens such as lettuce and spinach—benefits from a little extra moisture before refrigeration. Just don't use soap and hot water!

While root vegetables need a scrubbing with a brush to clean off dirt, other vegetables and fruits can be swirled through a basin or tub of cold water, dried off with paper towels, and wrapped carefully in more paper towels and plastic—and, of course, refrigerated. Even though veggies labeled as prewashed may be safe enough to eat without extra rinsing, why take a chance? Give them a quick rinsing and drying off. Rinsing and wrapping also applies to fresh herbs, even to the herbs picked from your own garden.

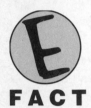

FACT

As a savvy consumer, you want to know more about keeping your produce safe; check out this FDA website: *www.cfsan.fda.gov/~dms/prod safe.html#stayinghealthy* or *www.fsis.usda.gov/Fact_Sheets/Seasonal_ Food_Safety_Fact_Sheets/index.asp.*

Cooking Methods

You are getting a meal ready, and now's the best time of all: cooking. Your ingredients, your tools, and you are ready to go. You may know all the basic cooking and cutting techniques, but there are a few things you are not sure about. Here are a few tips.

Adapting Your Recipes

You may live alone and cook for one, so adapting your recipes is not a problem, unless you are just starting on your vegetarian meal plan. Then you'll probably want to use the convenient soy meat alternatives often: these help keep you on track while offering you some familiar tastes and textures.

You might even try adapting some of your old-time favorite meat-based dishes to a vegetarian recipe—spaghetti and vegetarian meatballs will taste not much different from the dish you used to prepare—and friends and family may not even know the difference. You'll find plenty of meat-like soy products that will help make the vegetarian transition easier, and who knows? You could convince someone near and dear to follow along your vegetarian pathway.

But if you are the only vegetarian in the household, you'll want to negotiate how meals should come together. You'll need to ask for help in the kitchen when it comes to cooking meat, or at the very least, reach an amicable agreement among all parties concerned. On the way to your peaceful solutions, you can remind others that vegetarian eating is nutritious, colorful —just look at the range of colors on the dinner plate—and simple to prepare, as well as kind to the budget.

Basic Cooking Techniques

Here is a list of basic cooking methods and a description of each one:

- **Stir-frying:** The traditional Chinese cooking method calls for quick-cooking cut-up foods in a little oil over high heat while you constantly stir and toss the ingredients. Cook the densest vegetables first, the most delicate last. Correct stir-frying retains both the texture and flavor of the ingredient.
- **Sautéing:** Similar to stir-frying, sautéing quick-cooks foods in minimal amounts of oil; this is useful for larger cuts of vegetables.
- **Roasting:** Oven-roasting vegetables is a popular and effective way to slow-cook batches of whole or cut-up vegetables, either alone or combined with other varieties. To prevent drying out, vegetables should be tossed in minimal amounts of oil; flavoring the vegetables with herbs and other seasonings yields delectable results. This slow-cook method draws out natural flavors.
- **Poaching:** A low-fat way to cook vegetables, poaching calls for cooking a vegetable in a small amount of water or vegetable broth; you can season the cooking liquid with herbs, if you want. For uniform cooking, the vegetable or vegetables should be cut to similar sizes.
- **Steaming:** Adherents of steaming vegetables point out that this slow-cook method in which the vegetable sits above, not in, the cooking water retains nutrients and produces a crisp-tender result. The trick is keeping the steaming basket above the boiling water and covering the slow cooker so steam does not escape.
- **Blanching vegetables:** Blanching helps retain natural color lost in high-heat cooking. Just plunge vegetables into boiling water for

several seconds, and then plunge into ice water to stop the cooking. The outer layers soften without losing crispness. You can use blanched vegetables in salads and other cold dishes, add them to stews or soups, or finish cooking them in a stir-fry.

Slow, Slow Cooking

Not surprisingly, the versatile slow cooker can become a vegetarian's best friend. It can cook, roast, steam, and even bake, but obviously, it cannot grill. It lends itself to readying a wide range of vegetarian ingredients, from beans and lentils to root vegetables and grains. You can even slow-cook breads and desserts, all without your keeping an eye on the oven or the timer. Of course, as with any meal preparation, you will need to ready ingredients for the slow cooker. But then, it's just set the heat level, click on, and go—for several hours or for the whole day.

Plan Ahead, Cook Ahead

With today's busy lives, keeping ahead of the game saves your nerves and wear and tear on your energy. Before you head to market, check your shelves and refrigerator for all the missing items. Figure out your meal plan ahead of time, and make a complete shopping list so you don't waste time running out for missing ingredients. You might want to cook up several batches of some recipes; freezing made-ahead meals is a real timesaver. Batch cooking also saves on household energy, and cutting down on the costs of electricity and gas could mean real savings.

Basic Planning Tips

Everyday convenience cooking saves the modern consumer last-minute meal disasters—that means thinking about cooking ahead for those work-week meals when you won't have time for casual cooking. Before you cook ahead, however, you may want to stock up on plenty of tempting vegetarian recipes, either gathering a small library of vegetarian or vegan cookbooks, or printing out appealing dishes from a website.

You may also want to challenge yourself to get creative. If you have eaten at vegetarian restaurants, you'll know that the range of delicious vegetarian food is almost infinite. To get ideas, browse your local markets, even taking stock of their salad bar components, look for vegetarian groups in your community for recipe swapping and other good food ideas, and get online with a vegetarian chat room.

You'll want to stock up on solid containers with tight-fitting lids for storing the leftovers. This is particularly important if you are the frugal and organized cook who prepares and freezes several meals so you have good eats handy. You'll probably want to do that once you are comfortable with what fits into a vegetarian diet; making a week's worth of meals makes sense if you work long hours every day.

Cooking with Ease

As you get ready to cook, read through the recipe to be sure that you understand the techniques and, if you have a busy schedule, that you will have the time to complete the dish. Then prep your ingredients; this way, you can assemble the recipe without stopping to chop or measure. Other important do-ahead tips: Be sure to preheat the oven for baking or roasting, to grease a pan before baking, and to sharpen knives for easier cutting.

Celebratory Meals

Whether you are planning for a friend's party, a casual social gathering, or a full-scale holiday meal, you need to look at the guest list before you figure out the menu. You may have changed the way you eat, but maybe friends and family haven't. It's one thing to have your own beliefs and eating plans, but it's another to force others to follow along.

True, you could prepare smart and sophisticated all-vegetarian meals and mix it up with a sampling of ethnic vegetarian fare. Maybe people won't be disappointed that you haven't served a roast turkey or grilled some pork, but you could be a real crowd pleaser by offering a variety of dishes to satisfy everyone.

As for traditional meals, check in with family and friends beforehand. Ask someone else to prepare and bring the main-course meat, or if you are an invited guest, tell your hosts you will bring along your own all-veg entrée. It's that simple, and keeps everyone happy.

Don't Forget Snacks!

Are you one of those people who gets the afternoon snack attacks and really needs something sweet, fast? Do you dare to go shopping when you are really, really hungry, and end up buying way more than you can use or eat?

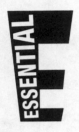

You can buy tasty trail mix combos easily, but why not make your own? That way, you can tailor the mix to include your very favorite ingredients. For a spurt of energy from your trail mix, include dried fruits, such as raisins, cranberries, and blueberries, and your favorite nuts and seeds. Store your trail mix in an airtight container, and watch the mix disappear.

You can make wise choices to keep hunger at bay by stocking plenty of fresh fruits, protein and energy bars, and some homemade choices such as hummus and guacamole that you can enjoy with chips or pita slices. Other tasty options for the afternoon—or morning—doldrums are freshly popped popcorn sprinkled with grated Parmesan cheese or herb seasonings; your own or a commercial trail mix; fruit-flavored yogurts; a black, kidney, or pinto bean dip with taco chips; and bananas or slices of whole-grain bread slathered with peanut, cashew, or almond butter.

CHAPTER 5

Starting the Day

Rise and shine! And then eat a sound, day-starting breakfast. Medical experts and researchers—and our moms—always remind people that eating a nutritious meal first thing in the morning revs up the metabolism, perks people up, and fosters clear thinking. Even late risers can linger over a wholesome meal, calling it brunch, and get an energy boost for the day.

Why Breakfasts?

Just about everyone has heard that eating a nourishing breakfast is the best way to start the day. Why? For one, your body has fasted overnight, and you need to refuel yourself. You also need an energy boost—not just a cup of hot coffee—to kick-start your metabolism and fully wake up. As an added incentive, a nutrient-packed breakfast—which doesn't need to be a buffet-style binge—sharpens your wits. After all, your brain needs energy, too.

Research suggests that people who eat well in the morning are less likely to overeat later in the day, a big bonus for calorie counters, who might be more inclined to skip breakfasts as one way to diet. Healthful breakfasts may also help you reach your daily levels of needed proteins, vitamins, and minerals while at the same time keep cholesterol levels down. Just make it simple and keep it fresh.

And good breakfasts are not just prescriptions for adult health: the American Dietetic Association notes that youngsters need to start the day off with a good meal—that way they can reason better at school and exercise more actively at play. All in all, then, eating a satisfying breakfast is a win-win game for everyone.

What's on the Table?

Planning out a balanced breakfast should be easy if you study the Oldways Food Pyramid or the USDA's MyFood Pyramid. With these guides, you will figure out the best sources of proteins, carbohydrates, and fats from the many options at hand.

Protein Portions

That all-important nutrient, protein, helps fill you up and squelches hunger pangs until lunchtime by helping to keep blood sugar levels up. For vegetarians who include eggs and dairy products in their diet, building breakfasts around rich protein sources is a snap: soymilk, whole or skim milk, eggs, yogurt, hard and soft cheeses like ricotta and cottage cheese, and grains and legumes are ideal day-starters. You can also turn to the numerous soy meat alternatives and the various types of tofu for real energy boosters.

For stricter vegetarians, getting ample protein is still a cinch: nut butters, tofu and tempeh, special grains and cereals, legumes, and soy meat alternatives fill the bill.

Kindly Complex Carbs

In the past, the words *starch* and *carbs* have become big headliners, adding to the confusion about what people should or should not be eating. Dieters, health food faddists, nutritionists, and just about every savvy consumer have weighed in on the carbs/no carbs debates.

But you should know this: Carbohydrates are essential elements in the diet. To get a handle on the debate, understand the differences between simple carbohydrates—the simple sugars found naturally in fruits, in vegetables, and in those products such as cakes and sodas made from refined sugars, for example—and complex carbohydrates, made up of fibers and starch found in all plant materials.

Complex carbs help the body to function smoothly, to regulate the digestion of sugars and the release of energy, and to keep at a balanced weight. Eliminating carbohydrates in favor of a protein-only diet, as some groups propose, can lead to chronic health problems. Note that besides starch and fiber, unrefined complex carbohydrates add vitamins and minerals to the diet.

Putting complex carbs on the breakfast table means serving whole-grain breads and cereals, plenty of whole fruits and vegetables, and/or cooked legumes. How about a baked sweet potato loaded with sweet or savory add-ins to start your day?

Essential Fats

With their negative connotation, fats have taken a bum dietary rap, yet everybody needs some dietary fats. And what to consume and how much are spelled out clearly by the Food and Drug Administration in its Dietary Guidelines, at *www.health.gov/DIETARYGUIDELINES/dga2005/document/html/chapter6.htm*.

Experts stress that you should avoid trans fatty acids by choosing fats and oils—olive oils, soybean oil, flaxseed oil, and nuts, for example—that contain no saturated fats or trans fats; limit the oil and fat intake to about 20 to 35 percent or less of your daily caloric intake; and routinely select foods naturally low in fat. Although vegetarians have cut out such fat sources as animal meats from the diet, you should also limit the amounts of cheeses and other whole-milk dairy products to keep your fat intake in check.

Breakfasts on the Run

Everybody does it—you grab a quick bite before rushing off to get to work, to school, to the train or bus, or to a meeting on time. And it's easy to miss out on the basics when you don't plan ahead for those super-busy days. But since breakfasts need to pack in the protein and complex carbs, you should stock up on quick bites that offer what you need.

Since grab-and-go options are plentiful, from microwavable entrées to ready-to-go whole grain cereals and granola bars, you can easily avoid the convenient fast-food eats that are high in calories and fats and skimpy on the rest of the nutrients. And in a pinch, you can pick up your breakfast at your favorite coffee shop, bakery, or fast-food outlet that serves vegetarian-friendly menu items.

Eggs and Egg Replacers

In and out of dietary and health favor, the egg—that perennial and ancient staple—has come back into fashion once again, with the added caution: in moderation. Why? Because recent research suggests that eggs have valid nutritional benefits for both the brain and the heart. The studies acknowledge that eggs do contain cholesterol, but that saturated fats, not cholesterol from eggs, may be a contributing factor for heart disease.

As a study conducted by the Harvard School of Public Health confirms, cholesterol from eggs and other dietary sources does not play a big role in heart disease, so it cautiously suggests that for most people, eating one egg a day is not putting them at risk.

Nevertheless, the American Heart Association recommends limiting egg consumption to four a week, and better yet, using the cholesterol-free white with 2 teaspoons of unsaturated oils instead of the whole egg for added protein intake.

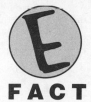

According to the American Egg Board, one egg contains seventy-five calories, plus various essential nutrients. For more egg information, check out *www.aeb.org/health_professionals.html*.

Benefit of Eggs

Besides providing an excellent source of protein, eggs—eaten in moderation—provide such needed nutrients as essential vitamins, iron, zinc, and lutein, a carotenoid that may help keep eyes healthy. And they are low in saturated fats.

Besides, eggs are easy on the pocketbook. They are also easy on the cook, for eggs can be eaten solo, whipped into numerous dishes, and added to baked goods, all good reasons to consider an egg as a protein option.

Not all eggs are the same, however, as you may discover in your dairy case. Not only do size and color vary, but also eggs may come from hens fed on diets enriched with omega-3s, hens allowed a free-range diet, and hens fed on organic foodstuffs. You can even find hens fed on a vegetarian diet, which means their eggs are naturally lower in cholesterol.

As with any fresh product, you'll need to handle eggs safely: check the sell-buy date on the carton; check that all eggs are whole without any hairline cracks on the shell; and refrigerate and cook eggs properly at home.

Egg Substitutes

If you are on an eggless diet, you need to consider other protein substitutes for the whole egg—and you have plenty of options to consider. Because you can chop, scramble, whip, or beat it, and it adds both texture and protein, tofu is an excellent egg substitute. For baked goods when you need added moisture, you might use a banana, applesauce, potato starch, mashed potatoes, puréed winter squash, or mashed cooked prunes as egg substitutes. Check your vegan cookbooks or recipes to figure out the egg-to-substitute ratio. But remember, eggs are also leavening agents, so you'll need to use an egg replacer or another ingredient such as baking soda or buttermilk to achieve a good baked result.

You can find powdered egg replacers at health food stores and many whole-food markets; to use them properly, follow package directions. But remember, egg replacers and egg substitutes do not cook up the same way eggs do, so you may have to experiment to get the results you are looking for. For more ideas, check out *www.foodsubs.com/Eggs.html*.

From the Dairy Aisle

Any food made from cow's milk is classified as a dairy product, and as you stroll along the dairy aisle looking at all the cheeses, yogurts, milks, creams, and butters, you can start planning some menus. Indeed, you could probably whip up a week's worth of dishes based on these fresh dairy basics.

You can expand your cooking repertoire if you consider such products as canned evaporated skim and whole milks; sweetened condensed milks; and powdered skim, buttermilk, and whole milks.

Because milk and its products are considered one of nature's almost perfect foods, its protein and high calcium content make it a desirable meal component. According to the USDA, Americans get nearly 72 percent of their calcium from dairy foods. However, some research shows a possible correlation between high milk consumption and the incidence of prostate and ovarian cancers.

Cheese Please

Because cheese contains many of milk's proteins, minerals, and fat-soluble vitamins, including cheese in your menu planning is a dietary bonus. Because it's an excellent source of calcium, cheese helps build bones and strengthen teeth, and might even help adults avoid certain health problems.

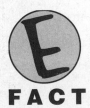

It takes ten pounds of milk to make one pound of cheese, says the National Dairy Council. That means, depending on the type of production process, that milk's many nutrients are condensed in a portion of cheese.

For children, cheese is a delicious way to add protein and calcium to their diet. But as rich as cheese is in protein and minerals, full-fat cheeses also have a relatively high fat and cholesterol content. So cheese lovers beware: moderation. Otherwise, stick to such lower-fat options as ricotta, part-skim mozzarella cheese, and cottage cheese.

For cooks, the charm of cheese lies in its versatility and in its range of flavors and textures. Cheese can work well in savory and sweet dishes, making it a desirable component for breakfast dishes, entrées, and desserts. And you can use its many forms: it crumbles, melts, slices, spreads, grates, cubes, and shreds.

Because of consumer demands for high-quality cheeses, many entrepreneurs have responded by initiating their own artisanal cheese makers' groups and relearning the art of cheese making. The result: artisanal cheeses that are produced in small batches, often by local artisans who milk their own cows and goats, produce their own cheeses, and sell them at farmers' markets. Fortunately, many fine artisanal cheeses are available online. Check out such websites as *www.artisanalcheese.com* and *www.artisancheesecenter.com*.

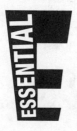

Did you know that people crave cheese more than any other food? That's according to the USDA, and in 2007, the U.S.'s cheese production totaled nearly 10 billion pounds.

Dairy Substitutes and Products

If you have eliminated all dairy products from your diet, you should consider such nondairy options as soymilk and the soy-based products, including soy cream cheese, soy sour cream, soy yogurt, soy margarine, and soy flavored cheeses. You'll also find in most health food markets nut-and-rice-based "milks." Whipped toppings and nondairy creamers are sold in most supermarkets. In general, dairy and cheese alternatives have no cholesterol, fewer calories, and less fat. For more information about soy-based, dairy-free products, check out *www.soyfoods.org/products/soy-fact-sheets/soy-non-dairy-alternatives*.

Yogurt and Your Health

Fermented and cultured milk products such as yogurt have been around for thousands of years, but they are easily one of modern man's most popular dairy items. Yogurt has a wide following in many countries, and it is appreciated by vegetarians and nonvegetarians for its health-promoting properties. Dieters also love yogurt in all its many flavors.

Among its many benefits, yogurt promotes longevity, some believe. Others eat yogurt because its beneficial live cultures of bacteria regulate the digestive tract and settle gastrointestinal upsets, aid the absorption of certain minerals, help reduce cholesterol levels, and may help prevent osteoporosis.

As with almost any food today, yogurt comes not only in many different flavors, but also with many different classifications. Whether you buy fat-free or whole-milk yogurt, look for one that is not heat-treated, contains active live cultures, and preferably is organic. For detailed yogurt information, visit *www.aboutyogurt.com*.

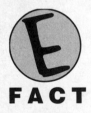

FACT

You can make yogurt cheese by draining plain yogurt, either the fat-free or whole-milk variety, in a cheesecloth-lined colander. The longer it drains, the thicker it becomes. Once it's as thick as you want, spoon it out of the cheesecloth and store it in a clean container. If you want, you can stir in seasonings to make it a sandwich or cracker spread. Otherwise, put dollops on your veggies, cereals, or cooked grains.

Veggie Frittata

Versatile and adaptable to whichever veggies are in season, this wholesome dish starts the day with a bang, and it makes a good light supper, too. It's easy to increase quantities to feed larger groups, so judge the size of your crowd. Made too much? This is delicious packed up for lunch. Offer plenty of hot coffee, hot tea, or hot cocoa and some fresh fruit.

1. Preheat the broiler.

2. Heat the oil in an 8- or 9-inch skillet over medium heat. Add the potatoes and sauté for about 3 minutes or until the cubes begin to brown. Add the asparagus, zucchini, garlic, and seasonings and cover the skillet, cooking for 2 to 3 minutes.

3. Meanwhile, beat the eggs until foamy. Stir in the cheese and parsley and pour the egg mixture over the vegetables. Using a spatula, lift up the edges of the eggs and tip the skillet to all sides, allowing the uncooked eggs to flow underneath the vegetables and to cook.

4. When the eggs are almost firm, slide the skillet under the broiler and cook until the top is bubbly and brown. Serve hot sliced in wedges; the cheese should be melted and runny.

What's Smoked Paprika?

A Spanish seasoning made from slowly oak-smoked and ground *pimentón*, a variety of Spanish red pepper, smoked paprika imparts an earthy, woodsy taste to an infinite number of savory dishes. It's readily available in well-stocked supermarkets, specialty food stores, and online mail-order sites.

SERVES 4

350 calories
23g fat
20g carbohydrates
16g protein
430mg sodium
2g fiber

INGREDIENTS:
3 tablespoons olive oil
2 red potatoes, diced
6 asparagus spears, trimmed
    and cut into 2-inch lengths
½ zucchini or yellow summer
    squash, diced
2 teaspoons minced garlic
1 teaspoon seasoning salt
1 teaspoon smoked paprika
6 large eggs
1 cup shredded Cheddar cheese
½ cup chopped Italian parsley

Hawaiian Turnovers

SERVES 8

390 calories
23g fat
40g carbohydrates
7g protein
800mg sodium
2g fiber

INGREDIENTS:

1 (8-ounce) package cream
   cheese, at room temperature
½ cup confectioners' sugar
½ cup crushed pineapple, very
   well drained
½ cup shredded coconut
½ cup sliced almonds
1 teaspoon vanilla extract
½ teaspoon salt
1 (16.3-ounce) package jumbo
   buttermilk refrigerator
   biscuits
Milk for brushing

Jumbo refrigerator biscuits make handy wraps for both sweet and savory fillings. Look for this product in the refrigerated dairy case at your market. You can eat these turnovers right away, but if you let them cool, then wrap and chill them for later use, these become tidy portable breakfast treats.

1. Preheat the oven to 350°F. Spray a nonstick baking sheet with non-stick cooking spray.

2. Beat the cream cheese and sugar together until smooth and slightly fluffy. Fold in the pineapple, coconut, almonds, vanilla extract, and salt.

3. Unfold the biscuit circles, one at a time. Roll them out on a lightly floured surface to about 5½ inches round. Put about 2 tablespoons of the filling mixture into the center of the circle and fold one side over the filling to the other side. Crimp the edges shut and brush the top with milk. Place on the baking sheet. Repeat with the remaining ingredients.

4. Bake for about 15 minutes, or until the turnovers turn golden. Remove from the oven and eat hot or set aside for later use.

Banana-Oat Bran Waffles

Use either a standard nonstick waffle iron or a Belgian nonstick one that makes waffles with deep indentations to hold pools of rich maple syrup. This recipe yields six Belgian waffle squares, or three rectangles, but the yield may differ according to the size of your waffle iron. Be sure to use very ripe and soft bananas so they can blend into the batter. Offer warm maple syrup, or other fruit syrup, and melted butter.

1. Preheat the waffle iron. Spray both surfaces with nonstick cooking spray.

2. Beat together the eggs, buttermilk, bananas, and butter until well blended and smooth. Fold in the flour, oat bran, baking powder, and salt, stirring until just combined and moistened; the batter should be stiff, not runny. Fold in the pecans.

3. Bake waffles according to the manufacturer's directions. Serve hot with extra butter and maple syrup.

What's Oat Bran?

Because it is so high in fiber, oat bran has become one of the darlings of the health food world and is often touted as one of the soluble fiber foods that help lower cholesterol levels in the blood. It's also a welcome ingredient in the kitchen for its cookability in cereals, baked goods, soups, and stews, adding some texture and a delicate nutty taste.

SERVES 4

470 calories
26g fat
52g carbohydrates
13g protein
430mg sodium
6g fiber

INGREDIENTS:
2 large eggs
1 cup buttermilk
2 very ripe bananas
4 tablespoons melted butter
  plus extra for serving
1 cup all-purpose flour
½ cup oat bran
2 teaspoons baking powder
½ teaspoon salt
½ cup crushed pecans
Maple syrup or other fruit syrup
  for serving

MAKES 8 (3½-INCH-ROUND) CUPCAKES

460 calories
28g fat
45g carbohydrates
10g protein
420mg sodium
3g fiber

INGREDIENTS:

2 (8-ounce) packages nonfat cream cheese, softened
4 tablespoons unsalted butter, at room temperature
½ cup sugar plus extra for sprinkling
2 large eggs
½ cup white whole wheat flour
½ cup all-purpose flour
1 teaspoon baking powder
1 teaspoon salt
1 cup dried blueberries
⅓ cup soy bacon bits, or to taste
Sugar for sprinkling

Breakfast Blueberry-"Bacon" Cupcakes

Crunchy soy bacon bits are versatile add-ins for many dishes, especially salads and omelets. In this recipe, the bits add an unexpected savory crunch.

1. Preheat the oven to 350°F. Spray eight 3- to 3½-inch-round muffin or cupcake tins and set aside.

2. Beat the cream cheese, butter, and sugar at medium speed until the mixture is smooth and creamy.

3. Beat in the eggs one at a time.

4. Beat in the flours, baking powder, and salt until smooth.

5. Fold in the blueberries and bacon bits. Spoon the mixture into each cup, filling it about ¾ full. Sprinkle a little sugar on the top of each cupcake before baking.

6. Bake for 30 minutes or until the tops turn golden. Cool for 5 minutes, then remove from the muffin tins. Cool the cupcakes completely on a wire rack.

Cupcakes Versus Muffins

What's the difference between a cupcake and a muffin? Strictly speaking, a muffin is a less-sweet—and sometimes a savory—quick bread that is eaten without frosting. A cupcake is a lighter, sweeter baked good with frosting and destined for dessert. But these "cupcakes" are a cross between the two—both sweet and slightly savory. And if you want to frost them, use whipped cream cheese.

Fruit-and-Cheese Quesadillas

Bland mozzarella is a perfect backdrop for fruit, and you can vary the fruit and jam according to what's seasonally available. These are knife-and-fork quesadillas, too gooey for finger food.

1. Spread 1 tablespoon jam on a tortilla and sprinkle it with ¼ cup mozzarella cheese and ¼ cup diced strawberries. Fold over the tortilla to enclose the filling. Repeat with the remaining tortillas, mozzarella, jam, and strawberries.

2. Spray the skillet with nonstick cooking spray and heat it over medium heat. Cook the quesadillas, one or two at a time, until golden on the bottom, about 3 minutes. Flip over and cook the second side until golden and the cheese has melted.

3. Top each quesadilla with a dollop of yogurt, a sprinkling of strawberries, and a dusting of confectioners' sugar. Serve hot.

SERVES 4

380 calories
16g fat
42g carbohydrates
17g protein
530mg sodium
3g fiber

INGREDIENTS:
4 tablespoons strawberry jam
4 (6- to 8-inch) whole wheat flour tortillas
2 cups shredded mozzarella cheese
1 cup diced fresh strawberries plus extra for sprinkling
4 tablespoons strawberry yogurt for garnish
Confectioners' sugar for dusting

820 calories
9g fat
113g carbohydrates
62g protein
770mg sodium
7g fiber

INGREDIENTS:

1 cup low-fat vanilla yogurt
½ cup powdered skim milk
2 tablespoons flax seed powder
2 tablespoons vanilla-flavored
*   soy protein powder*
2 tablespoons vanilla extract
1 cup chilled crushed pineapple

Morning Sunshine Smoothie

You can vary the flavors by using any favorite fruit in the same quantity, but make sure you use only a vanilla-flavored soy protein powder.

Combine all the ingredients in a food processor or blender and purée. Serve cold.

Baked Pasta Custard

*As a wholesome counterpoint to this rich brunch dish, offer
your family a bowl of freshly sliced oranges or grapefruit
segments, or whatever slightly tart fruit is in season.*

1. Preheat the oven to 350°F. Lightly butter a 2-quart baking dish and
set aside.

2. Beat the eggs until light and foamy. Beat in the ricotta cheese and
sugar. Fold in the orzo, almonds, cream, lemon zest, vanilla extract,
and lemon extract and stir until well combined.

3. Bake for about 1 hour or until the custard browns and the center is
firm. Serve hot or at room temperature.

SERVES 4 TO 6

380 calories
19g fat
39g carbohydrates
14g protein
105mg sodium
2g fiber

INGREDIENTS:

4 large eggs
*1 cup part-skim or whole-milk
ricotta cheese*
1 cup confectioners' sugar
2 cups cooked orzo
½ cup slivered almonds
½ cup heavy cream
1 tablespoon lemon zest
2 teaspoons vanilla extract
1 teaspoon lemon extract
Lemon curd for garnish, optional

SERVES 4

990 calories
49g fat
95g carbohydrates
43g protein
1750mg sodium
7g fiber

INGREDIENTS:

1 tablespoon olive oil
1 teaspoon minced garlic
1 cup soy "sausage" meat
1 teaspoon Cajun or Creole seasoning or hot sauce to taste
2 cups whole milk
3 tablespoons melted butter
4 large eggs
2 cups shredded Cheddar or Monterey Jack cheese
3 cups cubed sourdough bread
2 cups fresh blackberries or blueberries

"Sausage" Bread Pudding

Vary the berry topping to suit your taste by using raspberries, blueberries, blackberries, or strawberries. If these are not available, substitute 2 cups of your favorite seasonal fruits cut into small cubes. This dish is ideal for a leisurely family brunch.

1. Preheat the oven to 375°F. Lightly butter a 2-quart baking dish.

2. Heat the oil in a large skillet over medium heat and sauté the garlic for about 30 seconds. Add and crumble the "sausage" meat, stirring as you crumble, and season with the Cajun seasoning. Reduce the heat to low.

3. Meanwhile, beat together the milk, butter, and eggs until foamy. Stir in the cheese and sausage mixture. Put the bread into the baking dish and pour the milk mixture over the bread.

4. Bake the custard for about 45 minutes or until puffy and golden. Serve hot with the fruit topping.

What Are Soy Sausages?

Made from soy proteins, soy "sausages" are available as links or as a compact product packed in a tube. In the tube, the soy meat is easy to crumble and sauté like its pork sausage counterpart; alternatively, it slices easily and pan-fries like a patty. Look for soy sausage products in a refrigerated case displayed with other vegetarian and vegan ingredients.

"Sausage" and Grits with Country Biscuits

This vegetarian take on an all-time Southern favorite, a sausage-and-grits morning dish, has the same cheese and sausage richness without those extra calories.

1. Bring the water and olive oil to a boil over medium heat and slowly stir in the grits. Add the salt and thyme and reduce the heat to medium-low, stirring often.

2. After about 5 minutes of cooking, stir in the cheese, garlic, seasoning, salt, and pepper. Cook 1 to 2 minutes more and set aside.

3. Heat a skillet over medium heat and spray it with nonstick cooking spray. Brown the "sausage" slice on both sides. Meanwhile, split and toast the biscuits or muffins and place on serving plates. Put one sausage patty on one half of the biscuit and spoon the hot grits over both the patty and the second biscuit half. Repeat, using up all the ingredients. Serve.

SERVES 4

590 calories
34g fat
47g carbohydrates
28g protein
1010mg sodium
2g fiber

INGREDIENTS:
3 cups water or milk
2 tablespoons olive oil
½ cup grits, preferably stone ground
½ teaspoon salt
½ teaspoon dried thyme
2 cups shredded Cheddar cheese
1 teaspoon minced garlic
Creole seasoning or hot pepper sauce to taste
Salt and freshly ground black pepper to taste
4 slices soy "sausage" meat, about ½ to ⅔ inch thick
4 homemade or store-bought biscuits or 4 whole wheat English muffins, halved

SERVES 2

550 calories
34g fat
46g carbohydrates
18g protein
500mg sodium
4g fiber

INGREDIENTS:

3 tablespoons butter
1 tablespoon olive oil
½ cup corn kernels
¼ cup chopped onion
½ cup chopped red bell pepper
1 tomatillo, diced
½ jalapeño chile, diced, optional
2 tablespoons chopped black olives
1 teaspoon minced garlic
1 teaspoon taco seasoning
3 large eggs
½ cup whole or skim milk
½ cup all-purpose flour
Pinch salt
¼ cup salsa for garnish
½ cup chopped fresh cilantro for garnish

Tex-Mex Puffed Pancake

This easy-to-prepare breakfast dish can be varied to make it as spicy as you and your family like. It doubles easily, but then be sure to divide the batter between two skillets or two 8-inch cake pans. The butter must be bubbly hot before you add the veggies and pour in the batter.

1. Preheat the oven to 425°F. Melt the butter in an 8-inch or 9-inch oven-proof skillet.

2. Meanwhile, heat the oil in a large skillet over medium heat and sauté the corn, onion, pepper, tomatillo, jalapeño if using, olives, garlic, and taco seasoning for about 5 minutes or until the vegetables soften.

3. Beat together the eggs, milk, flour, and salt until smooth. Spoon the vegetable mixture into the oven-heated skillet and pour the batter over top.

4. Bake the pancake for about 20 minutes or until puffed up and golden; do not open the oven door during baking or the pancake will collapse.

What's a Puffed Pancake?

Whether you call this a German pancake, a puffed pancake, or a Dutch baby, this pancake puffs up dramatically and is much like a popover in its outcome. The pancake is an ideal medium for sweet or savory fillings and/or toppings. Most recipes calls for the pancake to act as the base for fresh fruits, confectioners' sugar, and syrup, but this version gives you a savory start to your day. It's real comfort food, and one you'll prepare often.

CHAPTER 6

Kids' Fare

Getting children to clean the plate is one challenge. Getting them to eat the healthiest foods is yet another. Parents can stack the cards in their favor by offering kid-friendly meals that are delicious *and* nutritious. That's easy once you know the basics, and besides, moms and dads can benefit, too. This chapter offers nutrition information for children of all ages, as well as tasty and nutritious recipes kids will love.

Nutrition for Infants

Experts agree that infants thrive on mother's breast milk—nature's ideal food for babies—and that babies do not need other nourishment for at least the first few months of life. While breast milk provides all the nutrients infants require, under the watchful eye of the Food and Drug Administration, manufacturers of infant formulas try to develop products that match breast milk quality. While they do a commendable job, they can't duplicate the antibodies naturally present in mother's milk.

Breast milk may be baby's best food, but moms who breastfeed need to keep up with their own special dietary needs—extra protein and calories—and calcium, plus specific vitamins and ample fiber in order to produce the most wholesome breast milk. Before the baby's birth, vegetarian moms who plan to breastfeed should brush up on how to choose the best diet for nursing the baby. It should be one that includes a variety of healthful foods, like tofu and other soy products, greens and whole grains, healthful oils, fruits and fruit juices, legumes and nuts, and fluids such as cow's milk or fortified soymilk. And meals should contain on average 1,800 to 2,220 calories or more a day to keep up a plentiful milk supply—and mom's energy. You may also need to take supplements. Your best bet: get advice from your doctor or a registered dietitian.

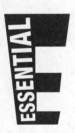

Not breastfeeding? That's no reason to skimp on your own meal planning. You may not need the same caloric intake, but you should still eat plenty of nutrient-dense foods. You've just had a baby, and your body needs to refuel itself.

While most experts—including the American Academy of Pediatrics (AAP), the American Medical Association (AMA), and the American Dietetic Association (ADA)—recommend breastfeeding, not every new mom can or wants to nurse. It's a very personal decision, and fortunately for new moms who decide not to breastfeed, the marketplace offers a variety of wholesome infant formulas. Most formulas are based on cow's milk; vegans should look for soy-based formulas but should first get their pediatrician to suggest the best formula for their baby's needs.

Feeding Youngsters

Parents make the ideal role models, especially when it comes to eating. If you set the example right from the start, odds are that your children will follow along. Show them that food—vegetarian food—is delicious, and that mealtimes are relaxed and enjoyable times. Just be sure you—and they—consume enough protein, fat, and calories to have the most energy throughout the day. For vegetarian parents faced with competing food temptations outside of the home, setting that early example is vital.

What Kids Should Eat

According to the American Academy of Pediatrics (AAP), your baby should be ready for solids between the ages of four to six months. By then, most babies have enough control over the tongue and mouth muscles to coordinate the activity of swallowing. The AAP offers parents some helpful guidelines for introducing solids—but be sure to get your pediatrician's advice as well. First solids should be easy-to-tolerate cereals, such as iron-fortified rice cereal, followed later by oat- and barley-based cereals, all moistened by breast milk or formula. Discuss the proper timing and foods with your pediatrician.

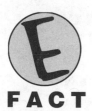

Just like your baby, your active toddler needs special foods to build strong bones and teeth. The Nemours Foundation states that a lacto-ovó diet with plenty of fresh fruits and vegetables and whole grains provides a sound nutritional foundation. See *www.nemours.org/e-service/kidshealth.html*.

By the time your baby is six to eight months old, you may, with the doctor's okay, start her on such protein-rich foods as tofu and cottage cheese and puréed legumes such as lentils. Vegetables such as puréed potatoes or sweet potatoes, green beans, or carrots come next, and bland and well-tolerated fruits such as ripe bananas, avocados, and applesauce help round out the diet.

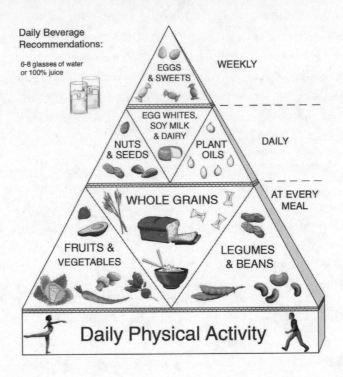

The Traditional Healthy Vegetarian Diet Pyramid for Children

Daily Beverage Recommendations:

6-8 glasses of water or 100% juice

EGGS & SWEETS — WEEKLY

EGG WHITES, SOY MILK & DAIRY

NUTS & SEEDS — PLANT OILS — DAILY

WHOLE GRAINS — AT EVERY MEAL

FRUITS & VEGETABLES

LEGUMES & BEANS

Daily Physical Activity

© 2000 Oldways Preservation & Exchange Trust, *www.oldwayspt.org*

By the time the baby becomes a toddler, at about one year, you might add cooked and mashed egg yolks and soy or dairy yogurt. As far as milk or a formula goes, the ADA suggests that one-year-olds should be offered full-fat cow's milk or a fortified soymilk. Infants or toddlers on a strict vegan diet may need extra supplements in their diet. Note that until your child turns two, you should not feed her a fat-restricted diet. Sources of fat can be unsaturated plant-source oils such as peanut and olive oils and the saturated animal fats found in regular cow's milk and cow's milk products.

Important nutrients for children include calcium and vitamin D for strong teeth and bones; iron for boosting red blood cells; zinc for cell growth and improving the body's immune system; and vitamin B12 for red blood cells and strong nerves. Vegan children may need supplements to meet their body's needs.

Don't Skip Breakfast

As it turns out, moms and grandmas were right: breakfast really is the most important meal of the day, for adults and most especially for children. Why? Everyone needs the basic fuels to start their metabolism revving up and keeping moods on an even keel. And researchers find that eating a nutrient-packed breakfast helps maintain a healthy weight, an important factor when so many youngsters are becoming obese.

The easiest way to serve wholesome breakfasts is to stock your pantry with whole-grain cereals, breads, and waffles; hard-boiled eggs; and ripe seasonal fruits. And for the mornings when everyone oversleeps, several eat-on-the-run treats such as yogurts, cheeses, or smoothies are great to keep handy. If late-rising happens often, try rousing the family earlier every morning, and the night before get the breakfast table ready; planning ahead prevents early-morning stress.

As you plan breakfasts—all meals, actually—keep in mind the balance between proteins, carbohydrates, and fiber. As a quick refresher, find your carbs in fruits, veggies, whole-grain breads and cereals, dried or cooked beans, and rice. Protein sources include eggs, cheeses, nuts, and dairy products. As for fiber, select whole grains, fruits, vegetables, and legumes.

Keeping Meals Kid Friendly

The trick to tempting little Susie to clean her plate is to offer foods she likes. Such standbys as noodles with vegetables or the classic macaroni and cheese options are usually sure-fire hits. For children without allergies, offer peanut butter with jam on whole-grain breads or baked into muffins. And burritos and tacos with cheese, soy meat alternatives, and/or vegetable fillings; pizzas; and dairy products such as cheese and yogurts are popular kid foods.

Still stumped? Try prepackaged veggie burgers or offer home-made bean or lentil burgers, and boost protein intake by adding meat substitutes such as tofu and soy "meat" products to soups and stews.

When planning children's meals, refer to the USDA's MyPyramid for Kids—omitting the meat option, of course—and use that as a general guideline. That means you'll end up with a daily diet based primarily on vegetables, grains, fruits, milk, and protein sources, with a minimal amount of dietary oils added for good measure. And ask your child to participate in meal planning: if she doesn't feel coerced into eating what you choose, chances are mealtimes will be happier.

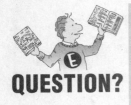

QUESTION?

Want to get mealtime cooperation?
Take your toddler on more than just a supermarket trip. Find a local farmers' market and browse through the stands, giving your child a positive experience with the glories of good, fresh foods.

Hungry kids—active kids—may need between-meals snacks, and instead of saying no, offer tasty treats that slip in extra nutrients. Why not suggest a crunchy apple or juicy orange, or perhaps whole-grain crackers with a cheese spread or hummus or a fruit-filled yogurt. Even a slice of cheese-topped pizza or a veggie hot dog will satisfy cravings. You can woo the young and hungry by keeping an ample supply of appealing and healthful snacks on hand: bowls of seasonal fruits, ready-to-eat veggies, and even bean dips with chips. But be sure to avoid fat-filled, high-calorie snack foods that don't satisfy—or build health. These just fatten. And skip the sugary sodas and fruit juices that tend to fill up rather than nourish. Remember, what's good for your child is also good for you.

Fighting Childhood Obesity

According to the Centers for Disease Control (CDC), childhood obesity in America has reached epidemic levels. Over the last twenty-plus years, it has increased at an alarming rate, almost fourfold in the twelve- to nineteen-year-old age group since the 1976–1980 NHANES survey. Well-documented health risks of childhood obesity include Type 2 diabetes, coronary heart disease and stroke, high cholesterol, cancer, osteoarthritis, and others. And overweight children are more likely to be overweight adults with the same health risks.

What are the causes of obesity? Studies suggest that a sedentary lifestyle and a high-fat, high-calorie diet are the main factors that add up to childhood—and adult—obesity. But active vegetarian children may run little risk of becoming obese: by avoiding fatty meats and fried foods, eating appropriate portions of nutritious foods, and keeping away from high-cal fast foods and snacks.

Vegetarian Teens

In a 2005 Harris interactive poll conducted by the Vegetarian Resource Group, about 3 percent of Americans between the ages of eight and eighteen described themselves as vegetarians. That's up from 1 percent in 1997, and other surveys show that about 40 percent of the teen population call themselves vegetarians. This proves that going vegetarian is no passing fad but a growing trend among young Americans.

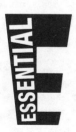

Like adults, teens give up eating meat and meat products for many of the same reasons—religious, ethical, health, and environmental concerns. There may also be some copycatting going on: several rock bands and movie stars are vegetarians, and may be inspiring their fan base to follow along.

Teens who opt for the vegetarian lifestyle must remember that just skipping meat does not add up to a vegetarian diet; they must plan meals that include the vegetarian basics: whole grains and greens, dairy products or fortified soymilks and cheeses, and fruits and proteins such as soy and legumes. They must also be sure that the foods they choose contain all the essential vitamins and minerals, with a special emphasis on calcium, iron, and zinc. That way they can make sure they stay energetic and healthy. Best bet: get nutritional guidance from a registered dietitian, and check out the website *www.vegetarianteen.com*.

Getting Going

Raising and feeding children is a challenge, but raising vegetarian children in a meat-eating society is a particular test for your vegetarian resolve. Problems will probably come up once little Susie is old enough for playmates and playdates and she gets offered a hamburger or chicken fingers by a well-meaning mom. Or maybe she helps celebrate a friend's birthday party and the group goes to a fast-food place. What is a mom or dad to do?

When you can, you should certainly tell others—from friends to child care providers—about your dietary preferences, but without making your child seem peculiar or freakish. And you can help your child make independent and healthful food choices when she is just beginning to eat solids, and continue to enforce right choices in the following years. By talking in an upbeat way about the foods you choose and the reasons you or your family is vegetarian, you can help instill the same attitudes in your child. Keeping mealtimes relaxed—and preferably, eating together as a family—underscores the pleasures of the table. And by permitting some food explorations, you will make vegetarian eating not seem forbidding and foreboding.

School Times

You may encounter more serious obstacles and objections once your child starts school. Despite the government's efforts through its National School Lunch Program (NSLP) to raise the quality of school lunches, many schools nationwide are still serving lunches and offering snacks that are high in fats.

But the good news is this: more school districts are making healthier choices, getting rid of offending vending machines, incorporating parents into lunchtime menu-planning decisions, and even offering some healthier choices and some vegetarian options such as salads on the menu.

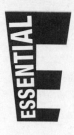

You can use the school lunch menu as an opportunity to reference healthy vegetarian eating and to make good food choices by reviewing it together with your child. Suggest selecting pastas, fresh fruit, salads, and whole-grain breads at lunchtime; even a slice of cheese pizza could be a wise choice. But if you feel unsure about how your child will face the lunch line or even how meat-free the menu options are, consider packing lunch instead.

The Vegetarian Resource Group writes that an increasing number of school lunch programs are including soy meat alternatives and vegetarian dishes more often on the menu. While economics plays a role in making these changes, at least some school districts view adding such vegetarian dishes as a way to improve child health and to meet the USDA's nutritional guidelines. Interested vegetarian parents can petition their schools to join in and follow these guidelines.

SERVES 4

300 calories
13g fat
27g carbohydrates
26g protein
2,200mg sodium
3g fiber

INGREDIENTS

*2 (7-inch) ready-made pizza
    shells*
6 tablespoons tomato paste
*2 Italian-style soy "sausages,"
    cut into circles*
*1 (4.2-ounce) package soy
    "salami" slices*
½ cup pitted Niçoise olives
*½ cup chopped pepperoncini,
    optional*
*Sprinkling crushed red pepper,
    optional*
Sprinkling Italian herb seasoning
*1 cup shredded soy mozzarella
    cheese*

Pizza with "Salami" and Italian "Sausage"

*A standard kid's treat goes vegan with this full-flavor pie. If
your child enjoys spicy foods, add the optional pepperoncini
and crushed red pepper, but with care. Otherwise, it may be
too hot to handle.*

1. Preheat the oven to 450°F. Spray the pizza shells with nonstick cooking spray.

2. Spread 3 tablespoons tomato paste on each pizza shell and place the shells on a baking sheet. Evenly distribute the "sausage" pieces, "salami" slices, and olives on each shell. Add the pepperoncini and crushed red pepper if using. Sprinkle the toppings with the Italian herb seasoning and cheese.

3. Put the pizzas into the oven, reduce the heat to 425°F, and bake for 5 to 7 minutes or until the cheese bubbles and the crusts begin to brown.

Pizza Shells
Most supermarkets stock premade pizza shells in varying sizes. Look for them in the freezer or near the dairy or bakery departments.

Cheese Dogs-in-Blanket

Resembling the old-time kid's favorite, Pigs-in-Blankets (hot dogs wrapped in dough and baked), these "dogs" are delicious with a side of hot vegetarian baked beans, sauerkraut, and plenty of relish and mustard.

1. Preheat the oven to 375°F. Spray a nonstick baking sheet with nonstick cooking spray.

2. Spray a skillet with nonstick cooking spray and heat the skillet over medium heat. Pan-grill the hot dogs until they start to brown all over. Remove from the skillet and set aside.

3. Lightly flour a work surface and roll out 1 slice of biscuit dough to about 5 inches round. Place 1 slice of cheese on top and put 1 "hot dog" and 1 tablespoon coleslaw on the cheese. Roll the dough around the "hot dog" filling and place this, seam side down, on the nonstick baking sheet. Repeat with the remaining ingredients.

4. Bake 5 to 7 minutes or until the dough turns golden. Remove from the oven, cool slightly, and serve with condiments, sauerkraut, and baked beans.

SERVES 4

520 calories
20g fat
52g carbohydrates
29g protein
1,720mg sodium
4g fiber

INGREDIENTS:
8 soy "hot dogs"
1 (16.3-ounce) package jumbo buttermilk refrigerator biscuits
1 (7.3-ounce) package soy cheese slices
8 tablespoons coleslaw

MAKES ABOUT 4 DOZEN COOKIES

Per cookie:
150 calories
5g fat
27g carbohydrates
2g protein
55mg sodium
2g fiber

INGREDIENTS:

1 cup unsalted butter, at room temperature
1½ cups firmly packed brown sugar
1 cup granulated sugar
2 large eggs
2 teaspoons vanilla extract
2½ cups white whole wheat flour
1 cup all-purpose flour
1 teaspoon baking soda
1 teaspoon salt
¾ cup chocolate chips
¾ cup jelly beans
¾ cup dried papaya cubes
⅓ cup dried cranberries
⅓ cup dried blueberries
⅓ cup pumpkin seeds

Trail Mix Cookies

These chunky cookies—packed with chocolate chips and other crunchy treats—will spoil your kids. The total "trail mix" add-ins may range between 3 to 3¼ cups. You can vary what you add to the mix, of course, but don't go over the total 3¼ cups.

1. Cream together butter and sugars until light and fluffy. Beat in the eggs, one at a time, mixing well after each addition. Stir in the vanilla.

2. Combine the flours, baking soda, and salt and stir into the butter-egg mixture. Mix until smooth, scraping down the dough from the sides of the bowl. If the dough still feels sticky, stir in extra white whole wheat flour, a few tablespoons at a time. Combine the trail mix ingredients in a separate bowl and stir them into the dough, making sure to distribute them evenly. Cover the dough with plastic wrap and refrigerate for at least 6 hours or overnight.

3. Preheat the oven to 350°F. Scoop out the dough with a heaping tablespoon for each cookie and place the dough on a nonstick cookie sheet. Repeat until the sheet is full, spacing the cookies about 1 inch apart; this should average about 12 cookies per sheet.

4. Bake the cookies for about 10 minutes or until the edges begin to turn brown. Let the cookies cool on the sheet before removing them and baking the next batch. Repeat until all the cookie dough is used up.

What Is Trail Mix?

Long-lasting and very portable, trail mix has become a favorite pick-me-up for those who enjoy rigorous activities such as hiking and camping. The mixture usually consists of such energy-dense foods as nuts, raisins, other dried fruits, chocolate bits, and granola and/or oats—a great energizer for kids! It's also called "scroggin" in such outback countries as Australia and New Zealand.

Sweet and Sour "Meatballs" over Brown Rice

This pleasing stir-fry brings together all the beloved flavors of a popular Chinese entrée, but instead of pork, you use kid-friendly "meatballs."

1. Drain the pineapple cubes and reserve the juice. Combine the juice, water, soy sauce, vinegar, sugar, cornstarch, and sesame oil in a mixing bowl, blending well. Set aside.

2. Heat the oil in a large skillet or wok over medium heat. When it is hot, add the "meatballs" and stir-fry for about 2 minutes.

3. Add the pineapple cubes, red pepper, zucchini, scallions, and garlic and stir-fry for 2 minutes.

4. Pour in the pineapple juice mixture and stir well to coat all the ingredients. Cook, stirring often, for about 2 more minutes or until the sauce thickens slightly. Remove from the heat and stir in the cashews. Serve over hot brown rice.

Vegetarian "Meatballs"

Although you can make a meatball-type product at home with a mixture of such ingredients as cereals, cheeses, and/or grains, most well-stocked markets offer in their specialty foods section heat-and-serve meatballs made from soy proteins. Kids—and adults alike—may never know the difference between these and the ground beef originals.

SERVES 4

670 calories
32g fat
76g carbohydrates
25g protein
1,690mg sodium
8g fiber

INGREDIENTS:

1 (20-ounce) can unsweetened pineapple cubes in juice
1 cup pineapple juice
½ cup water
⅓ cup soy sauce
¼ cup white vinegar
3 tablespoons granulated sugar
2 tablespoons cornstarch
2 teaspoons sesame oil
2 tablespoons vegetable oil
1 (9-ounce) package soy "meatballs"
1 red pepper, seeded and diced
1 zucchini, diced
1 bunch scallions, sliced on the diagonal
2 teaspoons minced garlic
1 cup cashews
2 cups cooked brown rice

SERVES 4

550 calories
13g fat
101g carbohydrates
13g protein
580mg sodium
11g fiber

INGREDIENTS:

*1 (28-ounce) can crushed
    tomatoes*
*1 (16-ounce) can or jar roasted
    peppers or about 8 roasted
    red bell peppers, skins and
    stems removed*
1 cup regular or soy sour cream
Italian seasonings to taste
Garlic to taste
2 tablespoons olive oil
*1 (16-ounce) tube polenta with
    sun-dried tomatoes*

Creamy Tomato Soup with Grilled Polenta Squares

*Kids love tomato soup with a grilled cheese sandwich, so why
not with grilled slices of polenta instead? If you want to, you
can always add the grilled cheese sandwich, too, for more
flavor and more nutrition.*

1. Combine the tomatoes and the peppers in a blender or food pro-
    cessor and purée until smooth. Add the sour cream, seasonings,
    and garlic and purée again. Heat the mixture in a saucepan over
    medium-low heat.

2. Meanwhile, heat the oil in a large skillet over medium heat. Slice
    the polenta into 8 circles and pan-fry one side, turning when the
    bottoms become browned. Turn over and pan-fry the second side.
    When both sides are golden and crunchy, remove from the skillet.
    Place 2 polenta circles in each soup bowl and ladle the hot soup
    over top. Serve hot.

Veggie Quesadillas

SERVES 6

300 calories
16g fat
27g carbohydrates
16g protein
670mg sodium
4g fiber

Most supermarkets now stock flour tortillas in several flavors, and this gives you a chance to use healthier whole wheat or multigrain options. You might even try out a flavored tortilla for a change of pace.

1. Preheat a large skillet or griddle over medium heat and spray it lightly with nonstick cooking spray.

2. Place 1 tortilla on a flat surface and sprinkle it with ½ cup cheese. Put about ⅓ cup vegetables and 2 tablespoons salsa on half of the tortilla and fold it over to close. Place the tortilla onto the griddle and heat until the first side turns golden and the cheese melts. Flip over to cook the second side. Repeat with the remaining ingredients, spraying with nonstick cooking spray as needed and not letting the griddle overheat. Cut the quesadillas into serving portions and serve hot.

Which Veggies?

These quesadillas are great vehicles for getting kids to eat their vegetables. Of course, offer their favorites, but why not slip in others, like radishes and sprouts? Head to your nearest salad bar and pick out a combination of vegetables, even pitted black olives and a three-bean salad, as fillings. Just make sure that the ones you select are shredded or sliced thinly enough to wrap up in the tortilla.

INGREDIENTS:

6 (8-inch) whole wheat or multigrain tortillas

2½ cups shredded Cheddar cheese

2 cups mixed shredded or cut-up vegetables

½ cup salsa

SERVES 1

480 calories
22g fat
48g carbohydrates
22g protein
430mg sodium
7g fiber

INGREDIENTS:
1 tablespoon olive oil
*1 tablespoon minced garlic, or
    to taste*
3 ounces soy "chicken" strips
¼ red onion, thinly sliced
1 10-inch flavored wrap
*3 tablespoons plain yogurt,
    preferably the thick Greek
    yogurt*
*2 tablespoons chopped fresh
    dill weed*
½ cup julienned cucumber
½ cup julienned red pepper

A Super-Hero Wrap-Up

*This is such a versatile carry-all for nutrients that you can
switch filling ingredients around to suit your child's palate.
While the filling ingredients are only suggestions, try to stick to
the amounts suggested, or the wrap may spill out all the
goodies.*

1. Heat the oil in a large skillet over medium heat. Sauté the garlic,
   "chicken" strips, and red onion for 3 to 4 minutes or until the onion
   wilts slightly. Set aside to cool.

2. Heat the wrap for 30 to 40 seconds per side in a nonstick skillet or
   according to package directions. Set aside.

3. Toss the "chicken" mixture with the yogurt, dill weed, cucumber,
   and red pepper. Spread the wrap out flat and top with this mixture.
   Roll up as desired.

About Wraps
You may use any kind of flat bread to make these portable sandwiches,
from pita bread to lavash, but most supermarkets stock flat breads—plain
or flavored—that resemble tortillas but are larger around. You must soften
these first before using, otherwise they may tear when you roll them up.
Follow package directions for rolling and folding, or simply roll the sandwich up like a tube and enjoy.

Breakfast Fruit Bars

Deliciously portable, these nutrient-packed goodies taste like a cross between a granola bar and a blueberry muffin, and the cream cheese frosting brings it all together. Note that you may use fresh or frozen cranberries in place of the blueberries.

1. Preheat the oven to 350°F. Butter and flour an 8" × 8" baking pan.

2. Beat the butter with the sugars until creamy. Add the eggs, one at a time, and beat well after each addition. Beat in the vanilla extract.

3. Stir or beat in the oats, flour, baking power, and salt until well combined. Fold in the blueberries and the almonds if using. Spoon the mixture into the prepared pan.

4. Bake for about 40 minutes or until the center feels firm, the edges are brown, and a toothpick inserted in the center comes out clean. Remove and set aside to cool. Slice into squares and frost with the cream cheese if desired.

SERVES 6

630 calories
24g fat
94g carbohydrates
11g protein
270mg sodium
7g fiber

INGREDIENTS:
¼ pound butter, softened
¾ cup firmly packed dark brown
  sugar
½ cup granulated sugar
2 large eggs
1 teaspoon vanilla extract
2 cups old-fashioned rolled oats
1 cup all-purpose flour
1 teaspoon baking powder
1 teaspoon salt
2 cups blueberries, fresh or
  frozen
½ cup slivered almonds,
  optional
Whipped cream cheese for
  spreading, optional

SERVES 6

440 calories
27g fat
37g carbohydrates
15g protein
730mg sodium
6g fiber

INGREDIENTS:
1 (1 pound) can pinto beans,
    drained and rinsed
2 cups shredded Cheddar
    cheese
1 cup crushed taco chips
½ cup salsa of your choice
½ cup sunflower seeds
2 teaspoons taco seasoning, or
    to taste
1 (9-inch) deep-dish unbaked
    pie crust

Taco Pie

*This wholesome entrée packs away all the kid-favorite flavors
of the Southwest—and the West—into easy-to-serve portions.
You can garnish each portion with guacamole, sour cream,
chopped black olives, more salsa for an extra kick, and
snipped fresh cilantro.*

1. Preheat the oven to 350°F.

2. Combine the beans, cheese, ½ cup taco chips, salsa, sunflower
    seeds, and taco seasonings. Sprinkle the remaining ½ cup taco chips
    onto the pie crust. Scoop the bean mixture into the shell, smoothing
    out the top.

3. Bake for 25 to 30 minutes or until the filling feels firm. Remove and
    set aside to cool slightly before slicing to serve. Garnish as desired.

Boosting Flavors
If your child likes taco flavors, use the opportunity to introduce other Tex-
Mex flavors. Maybe vary the cheese for a jalapeño bite, or check out
the Hispanic foods section in your grocery to come up with other flavor
options, such as tomatillos and different types of salsas.

Two Pastas with Three Cheeses

This dish lets you experiment with different cheeses, and depending on how adventurous an eater your child is, you might want to try fontina, Gorgonzola, or Asiago, or turn to more familiar cheeses like Cheddar, Swiss, or American cheese as one or more of the cheeses you use. The Parmesan cheese should remain, however.

1. Bring a large pot of lightly salted water to a boil. When the water comes to a rolling boil, add the pasta and stir once or twice to avoid clumping. Cook according to package directions, checking for doneness after about 7 minutes. When the pasta is al dente, drain and sprinkle it lightly with the olive oil, stirring to prevent sticking.

2. Meanwhile, heat the butter in a large saucepan over medium heat and when it has melted, add the flour and stir in the milk. Reduce the heat to medium-low and stir in the cheeses, mustard, garlic, and salt and pepper. Continue to cook, stirring often, until all the cheese has melted. Add the pasta, stirring well to coat it, and serve hot.

Pasta Shapes

These are only suggested pasta shapes; be sure to select pastas with ridges or indentations so that the pasta catches and holds the cheese sauce. Let your child pick out the shapes that he likes, too. Take him along and let him browse through the selections; you can even order some special shapes online.

SERVES 6

610 calories
26g fat
67g carbohydrates
26g protein
440mg sodium
2g fiber

INGREDIENTS:
½ pound dried orecchiette (ear-shaped) pasta
½ pound dried shells
1 tablespoon olive oil
4 tablespoons butter or margarine
4 tablespoons all-purpose flour
2 cups whole milk or soymilk
1 cup cubed Monterey Jack cheese
1 cup cubed mozzarella cheese
3 tablespoons grated Parmesan cheese
1 to 2 tablespoons Dijon-style mustard
1 to 2 teaspoons minced garlic
Salt and freshly ground black pepper

CHAPTER 7

Going Greens

Remember Mom's favorite mantra: "Eat your vegetables"? If you are one of the lucky ones who listened to Mom, you already appreciate how varied and delicious vegetables dishes are. It's easy to dress them up or to play it straight with a simple steaming or sautéing. And if you already have your favorites, move on to experiment with unfamiliar veggies and put your imagination to work. With so many choices heaped up in the marketplace, you have no excuse for not eating your vegetables.

The Benefits of Vegetables

Whether you want to lose weight, reduce your chances of developing certain cancers or chronic illnesses such as cardiovascular disease, or lower your cholesterol level, you'd better map out a diet that includes anywhere from four to thirteen servings of vegetables (including fruits) a day. As it is, most Americans eat perhaps as few as three such servings daily, making them very deficient in these beneficial foods.

While upping your vegetable intake may seem daunting, think of it as an exercise in coloring your palate: as the CDC points out, selecting vegetables —and fruits—in a rainbow's color assures you that you are getting the nutrients, including fiber, that you need for good health. That includes such multiple hues as red beets, white onions, blue blueberries, orange winter squash, and black beans.

Although using canned and frozen vegetables makes adding vegetables to mealtimes convenient and easy, shoppers should take advantage of growing seasons to sample everything from organic spinach to Asian long beans when these are stocked at supermarkets or farmers' markets. Fresh—and local—vegetables are often best. Like any living thing, plants have a finite life after harvest; greens are the most fragile and ideally should be eaten within a few days of purchase. On the other hand, sturdy vegetable like onions, potatoes, and winter squash last longer.

Important Health Findings

Do you still need convincing? Then consider the findings of the health experts about how valuable vegetables are for keeping fit. Researchers at the Harvard School of Public Health cited figures from a fourteen-year-long study of nearly 120,000 men and women and their dietary habits. The conclusions: Those who ate a diet rich in vegetables and fruits—about eight servings a day—had the lowest occurrences of stroke; reduced rates of certain cancers such as prostate and colon cancers; lower blood pressure and reduced risks of heart disease; better functioning digestive systems; and healthier eyes.

How to Up Your Vegetable Intake

Getting more vegetables onto your plate—or into your bowl—is really quite simple: for example, fold cut-up vegetables into a breakfast omelet; top your morning cereal with two different kinds of fruit; eat a salad for lunch *and* dinner; have fruit as a between-meal snack; top pastas with quick-cooked vegetables; put vegetables into such portable foods as sandwiches, tacos, burritos, and wraps; and blend fruit into a smoothie.

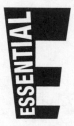

Vegetables and fruits are a reliable and natural energy source without hidden calories. Swapping vegetables and fruits for your higher-calorie ingredients—cream, butter, and loads of bakery goods, for example—helps you lose weight because most produce is low in fat and calories.

Leafy Greens

According to the USDA, *leafy greens* refers to such obvious candidates as lettuce, cabbage, chard, collards, kale, and spinach, but the category also includes broccoli—and all are members of the *brassicaceae* family with valuable cancer-fighting phytochemicals. The USDA also points out that there's good news for American consumers: their intake of these greens has increased by 9 percent, reports a CDC spokesperson of the period between 1996 and 2005. That's a plus for the health conscious, because as members of the crucifer family, the leafy greens contain cancer-fighting phytochemicals known as isothiocyanates. But scientists also warn that food-borne illnesses from improperly handled greens have also risen, which means consumers must be especially careful of how they handle their produce.

About the Greens

Ranging in shades from the pale lime-colored mustard greens to the darker greens of the chards and of collards, leafy greens are not only eye-catching in their natural beauty, they also form the muscle of a vegetarian diet: greens are easy to cook; they are extremely versatile, for they work as well in salads and sandwiches as in stir-fries and stews; and they have flavor profiles from pleasantly bland to sharp and biting.

Greens and Health

As nutrient workhorses, greens have few equals: most greens are loaded with vitamins A and C and certain minerals, including iron and folic acid. In fact, a 2004 study issued by Ohio State University confirms that the antioxidants in dark, leafy greens help ward off cataracts. Furthermore, researchers at the University of Liverpool in England found that eating plentiful greens reduces the risk of developing colorectal cancer, as reported in the June 2002 journal *Gastroenterology*.

Other studies conclude that leafy greens help lower blood pressure, aid in building stronger bones and healthier eyes, work as antioxidants, and protect against certain cancers. And yet another study suggests that eating more vegetables, particularly leafy greens, helps keep memories sharp, despite declines from normal aging. And of course, greens as a fiber source are excellent.

About Some Popular Greens

Today's supermarket produce aisles are stocked with numerous leafy greens for your eating pleasure. Some of the more popular varieties include the following:

- **Arugula:** Spicy, peppery arugula, also known as rocket, has long, tapered, dark green leaves. Good raw in salads or cooked in soups, and for pizza toppings or sandwich filling with other ingredients.
- **Collard greens:** A Southern favorite, collards with their long, sturdy leaves and rigid spines are a member of the cabbage family and have a mild, spinach-like flavor. Good for braising or steaming, enjoyed solo or stirred into soups, stews.
- **Kale:** The various kale varieties are members of the cabbage family, and the leaves have a slightly sharp taste. Its distinctive frilly leaves look relatively tough, but cook up quickly in sautés and in soups and stews.
- **Mustard greens:** A popular ingredient in Southern recipes, mustard greens have bright green leaves with ruffled or scalloped edges. Their pleasant peppery taste pairs well with ham or bacon. Steamed or sautéed, they are good as a side dish.

- **Swiss chard:** Available with white, yellow, or ruby red stems, Swiss chard has leaves that are large and veined and have a mild, spinachlike flavor. An elegant vegetable, chard cooks up much like spinach.
- **Turnip greens:** A cousin to kale and cabbage, turnip greens are also a popular Southern vegetable. The long, oval, crinkly green leaves are sweet when young but start to turn bitter as they age. They can be steamed, sautéed, and boiled and served alone or in combination with other greens.

Greens in the Kitchen

It's easy to convince yourself and others that greens can work well in your diet: they're best fresh and seasonal. Your best bet is to play around with which greens you and your family prefer. Remember that greens do need some beforehand preparation: Before cooking, rinse them well to remove any sand and trim off tough stem ends. Reserve the smaller, more tender stems and cook them with the leafy part.

Then experiment: braise, steam, stir-fry, or sauté (but don't overcook!) and season liberally until you find the method and recipe you like best. Don't be fooled by their bulk: One pound of greens cooks down dramatically, and offered as a side dish, may serve only two people.

Asian Greens

Thanks to the growth spurt in Asian restaurants and Asian markets in the United States, an increasing number of Americans can identify and feel comfortable with cooking and eating Asian vegetables, particularly leafy Asian greens. As members of the cruciferous vegetable family, Asian greens add both nutrients and interesting flavors to your family meals. And, in general, these greens are easy to work with and cook up quickly for a range of tasty dishes; some are tender enough to toss into the salad bowl without any precooking.

Because of their versatility, Asian greens are stalwarts in the Asian kitchen, maybe as revered—almost—as rice. Apparently, the Chinese are obsessed with eating greens: according to the Chinese news source, *People's Daily Online*, the average Chinese consumes about 311 kilograms of vegetables each year; the world average is only 105 kg. For more information about leafy Asian greens, check out *www.asiafood.org/asiangreens.cfm*.

Learning the Asian Greens Vocabulary

Asian greens—and Asian vegetables, in general—offer countless pleasures, but many may also bewilder the Western shopper who is unfamiliar with them. What adds to the novice shopper's confusion is that many Asian vegetables have more than one scientific name and several different marketplace titles.

For example, *bok choy* is also named *pak choi*; the long, white Chinese cabbage is commonly tagged *napa cabbage*; and *choy sum* is also known as *yu choy* and may be spelled *choi sam*. Then there's *tatsoi*, a variety of *bok choy*. And to mix it all up, many grocers use the general term Chinese cabbage to refer to numerous cruciferous Chinese greens.

If you just learn about a few of the basic and the most commonly available Chinese greens and vegetables, you can use that knowledge as a stepping stone into the glorious worlds of Asian foods:

- **Bok choy:** Full heads of mature bok choy, and its increasingly popular very young form known as "baby bok choy," are stalwarts of the Chinese wok. Although the very young plant is tender enough raw for a salad bowl yet captivating when stir-fried, it's the older plant that is more readily available. With its thick white stems and its broad, veined leaves, bok choy stir-fries well, producing a tender and mild-tasting vegetable that pairs with many different flavors and textures.
- **Napa cabbage:** Chinese, or napa, cabbage is perhaps the most familiar of Asian greens to Westerners. Its firm, compact, and lengthy form is comprised of white stems shaping into very crinkly, long leaves. Finely shredded for a quick stir-fry, the leaves also work well in soups and stews; if you have the patience, you can also substitute whole napa cabbage leaves for rolling up and stuffing as you would Western cabbage rolls.

- **Choy sum:** Resembling a cross between Chinese broccoli and bok choy, this lively green has long, slender, pale-green stems; tapering green leaves; and little yellow flowers. You can stir-fry it, but adding it to soups and stews adds color and a gentle flavor.
- **Chinese broccoli:** Also known as *gai lan*, *kai laan*, or Chinese kale, Chinese broccoli has long stems topped by dark green leaves and clusters of little yellow flowers. Cooks use the whole head, possibly peeling the outer layer away from tough stem ends, thus making the whole plant pleasingly tender. It's also popular in some other Asian countries, such as Thailand.

Sturdy Greens

Among the members of the vegetable kingdom, a small group of sturdy greens need the tenderizing effect of the cookpot to make them palatable and edible. But once cooked and ready for the plate, these veggies contribute both taste and some gastronomic diversions for the vegetarian—or for anyone. These vegetables include the artichoke; broccoli and the Italian, broccoli rabe (no relation); and Brussels sprouts, a mini cabbagelike green that most people love to hate.

Artichokes

A native of the Mediterranean and a member of the sunflower group of the thistle family, artichokes grow in selected temperate regions of the world. In the United States, they are the darlings of Castroville, California, a city that calls itself the "Artichoke Capital of the World." Baby artichokes, an early-summer star in the produce aisle, are just smaller versions of full-sized artichokes; these are often so tender they can be enjoyed with only minimal cooking.

Rich in nutrients such as potassium and vitamin C, mature artichokes do require trimming and cooking, and when tender, they are very versatile. They can be eaten solo or their very desirable hearts—once the choke is scooped out and the leaves discarded—lend themselves to a number of savory dishes.

Broccoli

An ancient vegetable that is a member of the cabbage family, broccoli is renowned for its health-giving benefits, particularly in its role as a cancer fighter. Although it is such a familiar vegetable and often an add-in to the salad bowl and to a stir-fry, some consumers may not know how to make the wisest choice at the market: for the freshest and best broccoli, select dark-green bunches with firm stalks and tightly closed florets. At home, broccoli should be refrigerated without rinsing. The hybrid broccolini comes from a cross between broccoli and Chinese chard, with the nutrient value and flavors that come from their parent plants.

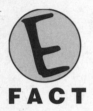

FACT

According to the USDA, one cup of chopped raw broccoli contains 31 calories, 2.4 grams total fiber, 43 grams of calcium, 81 grams of vitamin C, and 288 grams of potassium.

Broccoli Raab (or Rabe)

Also known as rape, rapine, or rapini among numerous others, despite its name this sturdy green is not related to broccoli, but is, instead, a member of the turnip family. It is sometimes called Chinese broccoli, which it closely resembles and some experts say the two are distantly related. With its little clusters of yellow buds on long, leafy stalks, it has an assertively sharp taste that adds character to soups, stews, and pasta dishes. The best bunches have crisp, bright-green leaves and clusters of partially opened florets on the stems.

Brussels Sprouts

Why these mini cabbages with their compact heads have earned such a poor reputation is puzzling. When handled and cooked properly to retain their crisp texture and pleasingly sweet-nutty flavor, Brussels sprouts add a spunky accent to any meal; they are even delicious cold when tossed into salads. The best sprouts should have dark-green leaves without any yellowing, and the heads should feel firm and compact. For cooking, the tough stem end should be trimmed away and any loose or yellow leaves discarded. Brussels sprouts steam, boil, sauté, or roast faster when sliced in half.

Roots and Tubers

Plentiful and easy on the budget, root and tuberous vegetables—from potatoes to beets to parsnips to sunchokes—fill many of the bins in the supermarket year round. Many, like the potato and sweet potato, are so popular that they turn up often on the dinner plate—and that's a bonus for vegetarians and nonvegetarians alike: roots and tubers generally offer few calories, no fat, some fiber, but many nutrients, depending on the vegetable.

Potatoes

Americans—and other nationalities, too—have a love affair with the potato, a starchy tuber that lends itself to frying, sautéing, baking, roasting, boiling, and steaming. Indeed, one source estimates that Americans consume about 140 pounds of potatoes each year. For potato facts and trivia, visit *www.npcspud.com.*

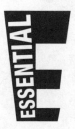

You may be interested to know that there was actually a potato magazine, published between 1917 and 1925. If you want to learn more about the romance and history of the potato, visit its virtual museum at *www .potatomuseum.com.*

Potatoes do supply some nutrients and fiber if you eat the potato skin. But while potatoes—which now come in numerous shapes and colors, some as small as thimbles and others darkly purple—are undeniably delicious, they are also an easily digested starch that may result in a rapid rise in blood sugar. According to the Harvard School of Public Health, potatoes and refined carbohydrates may play a role in the onset of Type-2 diabetes. So while you may love potatoes, especially if they are oozing butter and sour cream, you should eat potatoes sparingly, and more often substitute the sweet for the white potato.

Sweet Potatoes

A root often confused with the yam, a sweet potato is rich in vitamins A and C and, despite its sweet flavor, low in calories. According to the CDC, it is one of the most nutritious vegetables available. When shopping for sweet potatoes, select blemish-free ones and store them in the refrigerator, as they spoil rapidly at room temperature. Note that yams are tropical tubers native to Africa and Asia, and popular in African, Central and South American, and Caribbean cooking; true yams are not often sold in American markets.

Like the potato, the sweet potato is a multifaceted vegetable that may be cooked in many different ways. Baking it and eating it out of the skin is the easiest preparation. But the sweet potato may just as well be steamed, sliced and fried or baked, shredded raw before cooking, and whipped.

Mushrooms

Prized in many societies as much for their culinary as well as their nutritional benefits, although not a green, mushrooms can be a vegetarian cook's best friend. Versatile and nutritious—and low in calories—mushrooms can be puréed into creamy soups, rolled into burritos, and tossed into salads. But mushrooms, ironically, have some dark blots on their name. Why? Unless you are a trained mushroom expert, or mycologist, you can go mushroom hunting in the woods and just as easily pick a safe as a poisonous mushroom variety. That's why mushroom shopping at specialty food stores and supermarkets is the safest way to select these naturally nutrient-dense foods.

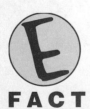

If you want to learn about mushrooms, spend some time browsing the website *www.mushroomcouncil.com*. It also welcomes mushroom questions if you cannot find the answers you want.

According to the USDA, the humble mushroom should not be ignored for the dinner table: mushrooms are sources of copper, potassium, and folate, to name a few nutrients. Asian studies of mushrooms suggest that mushrooms may help boost the immune system and may contain valuable antioxidants.

Mushroom Varieties

Years ago, the only mushroom readily available was the white variety, and that was often sold canned rather than fresh. Today's markets, however, offer consumers many of the thousands of wild and cultivated mushroom varieties. Look for such mushrooms as chanterelle, oyster, shiitake, enoki, portobello, cremini, maitake, and the very pricey morel at your market. In your Asian market, look for several dried varieties, such as the shiitake and the straw mushrooms.

Besides the popular white or button mushrooms, the very versatile portobello mushroom may be the consumer's top pick. Not only is the portobello a fine protein source, its dense, chewy texture makes for pleasurable eating. Because its cap may be large enough to replace a slice of bread, the portobello makes a delicious sandwich, and it can be grilled, roasted, stir-fried, and eaten raw.

420 calories
26g fat
28g carbohydrates
27g protein
1,190mg sodium
12g fiber

INGREDIENTS:

2 tablespoons olive oil
1 large onion, thinly sliced
1 (12-ounce) package Kielbasa
*   soy "sausage," thinly sliced*
1 bunch chard, rinsed and
*   coarsely chopped*
1 bunch collards, rinsed and
*   julienned*
½ cup grated Parmesan cheese

Sautéed Mixed Greens with Kielbasa "Sausage"

Bursting with flavor and nutrients, this greens medley suits a casual dinner; offer this with a toasted baguette.

1. Heat the oil in a large stockpot over medium heat and sauté the onion and "sausage" slices until the onion turns golden.

2. Add the greens and a sprinkling of water, cover the stockpot, and steam the greens until they are wilted and tender. Sprinkle the greens with the Parmesan cheese and serve.

Baked Spinach Tart

Popeye loved his spinach from a can, but you will love it fresh with its bright flavor and color.

1. Preheat the oven to 350°F.

2. Beat the eggs until foamy. Stir in the yogurt, feta cheese, mozzarella cheese, spinach, and onions, mixing well until combined. Season with salt and pepper.

3. Spoon the mixture into the pie shell and push the tomatoes into the top of the mixture.

4. Bake for about 40 minutes or until the mixture is firm to the touch. Let it cool slightly before slicing and serving.

SERVES 4 TO 6

490 calories
33g fat
28g carbohydrates
24g protein
920mg sodium
3g fiber

INGREDIENTS:

2 large eggs
1 cup plain nonfat or whole milk yogurt
1 cup feta cheese
1 cup shredded mozzarella cheese
1 bunch fresh spinach, preferably organic, well rinsed, wilted, and chopped
½ cup chopped onion
Salt and freshly ground black pepper to taste
1 (9-inch) unbaked deep-dish pie shell
½ pint grape tomatoes

SERVES 6

220 calories
16g fat
13g carbohydrates
9g protein
470mg sodium
2g fiber

INGREDIENTS:

2 tablespoons olive oil
4 cloves garlic, crushed and
    chopped
1 onion, diced
1 red bell pepper, seeded and
    diced
1 (13.75-ounce) can artichoke
    hearts, drained and
    quartered
1 sheet puff pastry, thawed
½ cup chopped Niçoise olives
3 tablespoons capers
4 ounces goat cheese, cut into
    cubes

Mediterranean Galette with Goat Cheese

You can add more capers and goat cheese, if you want.

1. Preheat the oven to 375°F.

2. Heat the oil in a large skillet over medium heat and sauté the garlic and the onion for about 3 minutes. Add the pepper and artichoke hearts and continue cooking until the onion begins to brown. Set aside.

3. Lightly flour a work surface and roll out the dough until it is about 10 inches long. Fit it into a 3-quart baking dish with the dough going up the sides. Spoon the onion mixture into the crust, sprinkle the filling with the olives and capers, and put the cubes of cheese on the top. Fold the pointed ends in toward the center, partially enclosing the filling.

4. Bake the tart for about 40 minutes or until the crust becomes puffy and golden. Serve hot.

What Is a Galette?

In France, the word *galette* can mean a flat bread or, as in this case, an open-faced and free-form tart. Fillings may be either sweet or savory.

Fiery Indian Potatoes

This unusual potato dish is not for the faint of heart, for the chili component can singe your eyebrows. Yet it is a delicious dish and pairs well with thick plain yogurt or as an accompaniment to other vegetarian dishes. Look for the Indian red chili powder at an Indian market; otherwise, use ground cayenne.

1. Steam the potato cubes until just tender. Set aside.

2. Heat the oil in a large skillet or wok, and sauté the potatoes for 2 minutes. Add the chiles, mustard seeds, turmeric, chili powder, salt, and pepper and continue cooking over medium heat, stirring, until the seasonings are well mixed and the potatoes begin to brown. Stir in the coriander, garnish with the cilantro, and serve.

SERVES 6

370 calories
8g fat
69g carbohydrates
9g protein
30mg sodium
9g fiber

INGREDIENTS:

6 large potatoes, peeled and cubed
3 tablespoons vegetable oil, or more as needed
5 dried red chiles, or to taste, crushed
1 tablespoon mustard seeds
1 teaspoon ground turmeric
1 teaspoon red chili powder
Salt and freshly ground black pepper to taste
1 tablespoon ground coriander
1 cup chopped fresh cilantro for garnish

SERVES 2

1,010 calories
38g fat
156g carbohydrates
24g protein
170mg sodium
17g fiber

INGREDIENTS:
½ cup pomegranate juice
1 teaspoon butter
1 cup uncooked couscous
¾ cup toasted pine nuts
10 dried apricots, coarsely
    chopped
½ cup cilantro leaves
Pinch salt
2 very large globe artichokes,
    trimmed and cooked

Artichokes Stuffed with Couscous

*Garlic mayonnaise is good for dipping the leaves and
seasoning the artichoke bottoms after the couscous is eaten.*

1. Combine 1 cup water and the pomegranate juice in a saucepan and heat to boiling, then stir in the butter and couscous. Remove from the heat and cover; set aside for 5 minutes.

2. Meanwhile, in a mixing bowl, combine the pine nuts, apricots, cilantro leaves, and salt, stirring well. Fold in the couscous.

3. Part the artichoke leaves to expose the center. Using a spoon, scoop out the central thistles, or choke, and discard. Spoon the couscous mixture into the artichokes, mounding it up to fill them completely. Serve hot or at room temperature.

Southwestern Sprouts

Don't turn up your nose at Brussels sprouts, especially when these are kicked up a notch with seasonings and texture. You'll want to serve these often.

1. Preheat the oven to 350ºF.

2. Toss the sprouts with the oil and taco seasoning and put them in a roasting pan. Cook for about 30 minutes or until the sprouts become tender.

3. Put them in a serving bowl and toss with the taco chips, salsa, cheese, and sunflower seeds if using. Serve hot.

SERVES 4

390 calories
24g fat
35g carbohydrates
14g protein
680mg sodium
8g fiber

INGREDIENTS:

1 pound Brussels sprouts, trimmed and halved
1 tablespoon olive oil
1 tablespoon taco seasoning or to taste
½ cup crushed spicy taco chips
½ cup spicy or mild salsa
½ cup shredded Cheddar cheese
½ cup sunflower seeds, optional

Overly Stuffed Baked Sweet Potato

SERVES 1

940 calories
49g fat
75g carbohydrates
53g protein
2,510mg sodium
16g fiber

INGREDIENTS:

1 large sweet potato
½ cup mild or hot salsa
¾ cup grated Cheddar cheese
1 jalapeño chile, diced, or more to taste, optional
½ cup cubed Monterey Jack cheese
1 cup vegetarian chili
Chopped fresh cilantro for garnish

To reduce calories in this robust dish, use reduced-fat cheese. And for even more flavor, you may increase the amount of salsa, or select one of the types that now include fruit and other interesting add-ins.

1. Bake the sweet potato in a 350°F oven until tender. Remove from the oven and, when it is cool enough to handle, slit open the top and scoop out the flesh, leaving a thin layer of flesh around the interior.

2. Mix the sweet potato flesh with the salsa, grated cheese, and jalapeño, if using. Spoon it back into the skin and dot the top with the Monterey Jack cheese. Return the sweet potato to the oven to cook until the cheese melts.

3. Meanwhile, heat the chili, and when the cheese has melted, put the sweet potato on a serving plate and spoon the chili over top. Garnish with the cilantro and enjoy.

Curried Sunchokes, Plantain, and Apples

Sunchokes and plantains do not make frequent appearances at the American table, but here they make a gentle trio with the all-American apple adding its own sweetness. With the addition of curry and ginger, this simple dish becomes an international star. An accompanying dish of cooked white or brown rice would balance out the meal.

1. Heat the oil in a large skillet over medium heat. Add the onion, ginger, and garlic and sauté for 2 to 3 minutes. Stir in the turmeric and curry and cook 2 to 3 minutes more. Add the sunchokes, apple, and plantain and stir until the mixture is coated with the seasoning.

2. Stir in the vegetable broth, reduce the heat to medium-low, and cover, cooking for about 10 minutes more or until the sunchokes are just tender. Stir in the peanuts and serve.

About Sunchokes

Native to North America and once a staple for some Native American tribes, the sunchoke—also called a Jerusalem artichoke—is not an artichoke but instead a tuber from the sunflower family; it resembles an oddly shaped small potato. Its crunchy texture resembles that of water chestnuts. These may be cooked or eaten raw.

SERVES 2

780 calories
41g fat
99g carbohydrates
18g protein
430mg sodium
13g fiber

INGREDIENTS:

3 tablespoons vegetable oil, or more as needed
1 onion, thinly sliced
2 to 3 tablespoons grated fresh ginger
4 cloves garlic, lightly crushed
2 teaspoons ground turmeric
1 teaspoon curry powder, or to taste
1 pound sunchokes (Jerusalem artichokes), scrubbed and thinly sliced
1 firm cooking apple, cored and thinly sliced
1 firm yellow plantain, peeled and thinly sliced
1 cup vegetable broth
½ cup salted peanuts

310 calories
21g fat
21g carbohydrates
15g protein
310mg sodium
6g fiber

INGREDIENTS:

2 cups broccoli florets,
    parboiled
2 cups chopped broccoli rabe,
    parboiled
2 cups chopped Chinese
    broccoli, parboiled
4 cloves garlic, chopped
1 cup toasted walnuts
½ cup crumbled Gorgonzola
    cheese
Balsamic salad dressing, as
    desired
Salt and fresh ground black
    pepper to taste
Crushed red pepper to taste

Chilled Broccoli Trio

*To parboil the broccolis, plunge each batch into boiling water
from 3 to 5 minutes, depending on the variety. Rinse each
batch under cold running water and drain very well.*

1. Combine the three broccolis in a mixing bowl and toss with the garlic. Chill until ready to serve.

2. Just before serving, add the walnuts, cheese, dressing, salt, pepper, and crushed red pepper. Toss well.

Stuffed Portobello Mushroom

The meaty flavor and texture of the Portobello mushroom make a great foil for a variety of toppings, including even dried fruits such as raisins, cranberries, and blueberries that accent a pasta or rice mixture as filling.

1. Preheat the oven to 375°F. Lightly oil a baking dish.

2. Combine the orzo, tomato sauce, mozzarella cheese, tomato, oregano, salt, and pepper in a small mixing bowl. Brush the portobello on the cap and the underside with olive oil. Mound the mixture in the center and place the mushroom in the baking dish.

3. Bake for 25 to 30 minutes or until the cheese has melted and the mushroom feels tender.

Cleaning a Portobello Mushroom

As with any mushroom variety, portobellos do not need rinsing, simply a wipe-off with a moist paper towel. Then carefully twist off the mushroom's stem. You may also want to remove the black gills under the cap. To do this, use a spoon and gently scrape them away. The gills impart a dark color to any surrounding liquids.

SERVES 1

680 calories
15g fat
107g carbohydrates
33g protein
750mg sodium
10g fiber

INGREDIENTS:

1 cup cooked orzo
½ cup tomato sauce
½ cup shredded mozzarella cheese
1 tomato, chopped
1 teaspoon dried oregano
Salt and freshly ground black pepper
1 large Portobello mushroom
olive oil for brushing

CHAPTER 8

Beans, Nuts, Lentils, and Chickpeas

For vegetarians, such protein powerhouses as legumes—beans and lentils—and nuts are the foundation of an all-veg menu, for these foods contain not only protein, good carbs, fiber, and micronutrients, they also, in the case of nuts, add some good-for-you fats. And for ease of cooking, these can't be beat. Almost every legume comes precooked in a can, and nuts are sold roasted and shelled ready for the breakfast, lunch, or dinner plate.

Why Legumes?

When you look at the class of vegetables known as legumes, you'll realize that these world-class foods are just that: universal favorites in practically every cuisine and welcome and healthful additions to everyone's meals. But just exactly what is this fabulous food known as a legume?

A member of the *Fabaceae* family, a legume is simply a dried fruit of these plants—alfalfa, beans, and peas, plus many others—that forms a pod, which splits in half along a seam. Inside, forming a single row are its seeds, such as beans, peas, and lentils; these are also known as pulses. Pulses are allowed to dry in the pod before or after shelling, but either way, are rehydrated in some form of liquid for use on the table. Some estimates suggest that about 18,000 species of legumes exist.

As important to man's diet as the greens and grains, legumes have been consumed for the past 20,000 years, with evidence of their consumption dating back to ancient Egypt and Greece and in South America for probably about 5,000 years. Historically, then, for much of the world, beans—legumes—have been a vital protein source.

Health Benefits

As a valuable source of protein, few foods can equal what legumes have to offer. According to the Linus Pauling Institute at Oregon State University, legumes not only provide protein, they also supply micronutrients, minerals, fiber, and good carbs. The institute points out that one study shows that patients on a legume-rich diet were 21 percent less likely to develop coronary heart disease than were those who ate legumes less than once a week.

Certain beans also contain disease-fighting antioxidants that might reduce the risk of certain cancers. And as the USDA notes, for vegetarians who exclude all animal flesh from their diet, legumes are an important protein source. Note that legumes contain little fat and no cholesterol, making them important elements for heart health and weight management.

How many servings of legumes a week? According to the USDA's 2005 Dietary Guidelines, people who eat on average 2,000 calories a day should include six servings—about ½ cup of cooked legumes, including tofu—a week. For vegetarians needing to up their protein, the intake should probably be higher. For more information, refer to *www.health.gov/dietaryguide lines/dga2005/document/html/chapter2.htm.*

The World of Beans

Today's markets have gone into offering dried and canned legumes in a big way, and varieties once uncommon—cranberry beans, field peas, and the French flageolets, for example—are relatively easy to find. The challenge for the vegetarian cook is coming up with enough ways to cook and serve these often bright and colorful legumes. Fortunately, legumes are easy on the pocketbook, so cooks can feel comfortable in their explorations and can more readily add beans to their diet.

And if you want to increase your bean intake, you can be proactive: try bean or pea soups; toss beans and peas into salads; mash them for a sandwich filling; try them as an omelet filling; or explore the numerous world cuisines that rely on beans as a kitchen staple.

Dried Versus Canned

Any way you look at it, eating beans, whether dried or out of the can, is an inexpensive way to enjoy a meal—of course, opting for dried beans costs only pennies per serving, since a one-pound bag of dried beans, or about 2 cups, equals about 6 cups of cooked beans.

But in the bean world, bean-eaters often join in the debate about using canned versus dried beans. Obviously, canned beans are faster to use, but many brands are packed with extra sodium, making these canned beans less desirable. To avoid excess sodium, you should buy beans that say "no salt added" or drain and thoroughly rinse the canned beans before using them. On the other hand, devotees of dried beans insist that these have a fuller, richer bean flavor.

Easy Prep Steps

If you prefer to use dried beans, remember that readying them requires planning ahead: dried beans should soak for at least four hours, but preferably overnight. Some sources suggest that lengthy soaking results in a creamier cooked bean. You could also boil them for about an hour in their rinse water, then drain them and cook them in plenty of water to cover. Finally, you could cook them in a pressure cooker, but definitely follow manufacturer's directions.

Many people have problems with beans causing gas and bloating, and thus, they avoid eating them. But you can try several measures to sidestep that problem: introduce beans into your diet slowly; cook them with a pinch of baking soda; and don't cook beans in their soaking water.

Note that the FDA warns that eating undercooked beans—particularly red kidney beans—can result in some unpleasant symptoms, including nausea and vomiting. Undercooked beans contain a substance called "lectin," a compound that, among other things, interferes with cellular metabolism. The symptoms pass quickly, but can be totally avoided by boiling the beans you eat.

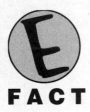

FACT

You can purée cooked beans easily by mashing them with the back of a wooden spoon or a potato masher, by pushing them through a food mill, or by whirring them in a food processor or blender. These purées are easy to enhance with oil or butter and to season with citrus juices, herbs, spices, or flavor accents such as garlic or ginger.

Nuts about Nuts . . . and Seeds

So you like to grab a handful of nuts and seeds between meals or at a party? What were once considered fatty and fattening foods, particularly nuts, have claimed a leading role in promoting good health—that is, if eaten in moderation. That's good news, especially for the cook: nuts and seeds are extremely versatile, and lend both texture and flavor to stews, sandwiches, desserts, soups, and stews, plus many other recipes.

If you've enjoyed those many handfuls of nuts, you may think you know what they are. According to *Merriam Webster's Collegiate Dictionary* (tenth edition), a nut is a "hard-shelled dried fruit or seed with a separable rind or shell and interior kernel." If that's a bit confusing, just remember that all nuts are actually seeds, but all seeds—for example, the tiny seeds encased in a blueberry—are not necessarily nuts.

Nutty about Health

Researchers chime in on this: nuts are good for you! In 2006 the USDA published a report of research that shows that because nuts—from Brazil nuts, cashews, and hazelnuts, to pecans—are rich in phytochemicals, they actually protect against heart disease, diabetes, and certain cancers. Besides, nuts are rich in both vitamins and minerals.

According to studies conducted by the Harvard Medical School and the Harvard School of Public Health looking at how eating nuts affects heart health, men who regularly incorporate nuts into their diet can reduce the risk of heart disease. The researchers concluded that nuts contain the heart-healthy mono- and polyunsaturated fats, omega-3 fats, and arginine, all of which play a key role in benefiting the heart and keeping it healthy. But because nuts are calorie rich, people should cut way back on other fatty foods, keeping their nut intake to about one ounce a day, according to the FDA; see *www.hsph .harvard.edu/nutritionsource/what-should-you-eat/nuts-for-the-heart*. Nuts on the A list include almonds, cashews, peanuts, pistachios, and walnuts.

The Harvard University Nurses' Health Study indicates that women also benefit by including nuts in their diet. Of the 84,000 nurses studied for several decades, those who ate at least one ounce of nuts five times a week had a 27 percent lower chance of developing type 2 diabetes than those who rarely if ever ate nuts. Those whose nut intake came only from peanut butter still were less likely to develop the disease. The study took into account age, family history, and body mass index. Harvard researchers also state that regularly consuming nuts helps cut the risk of heart attacks or cardiovascular disease.

For more about nuts and your health, visit *www.mayoclinic.com/ health/nuts/HB00085.*

Superstar Walnuts

In bygone eras, folklore relates, healers used walnuts for muscle aches and upset stomachs, and as a calming brain food that also boosted the IQ. But today's scientists are evaluating the walnut for its possibilities of promoting heart health.

In 2006, the USDA published a report stating that walnuts not only reduce the bad cholesterol, they also may help reduce plaque buildup in the arteries. For the study, researchers used the English walnut ground to a meal and fed to hamsters, all of which had notably lower levels of a compound that causes plaque buildup. Presumably, walnuts will have the same positive benefits for human heart health. Whatever their health benefits may be, walnuts are full of fiber and health-promoting fatty acids.

For more information about other walnut research projects, go to *www .walnutinfo.com/healthStudies.aspx*.

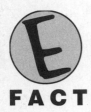

FACT

According to the California Walnut Commission, humankind has been enjoying walnuts since 7000 B.C. Walnuts have played other roles in history: according to the Commission, Michelangelo used walnut oil when he painted the Sistine Chapel.

Toasting Nuts and Seeds

As with most foods, heating draws out and intensifies the inherent flavors in nuts and seeds. But both must be watched carefully because they heat up fast and can scorch. To toast whole nuts or seeds in a preheated 350°F oven, place them in a single layer on an ungreased sheet or pan for about 5 minutes, stirring several times. Remove them from the oven, and cool on a second sheet or pan.

To toast them on the stovetop, the same principle applies: moderate heat, single layer in a skillet, no oil or fat, and frequent stirring. Cool them in a separate pan. However you toast them, smaller seeds cook faster, so watch them carefully. Store unused nuts and seeds in an airtight container in the refrigerator for up to two weeks.

Looking for Lentils

In the words of the late, beloved food writer Laurie Colwin, lentils are friendly beans, and it's easy to see why they have gained such an avid following. Lentils are packed with protein and fiber and contain ample amounts of iron, B vitamins, and folate. Besides these health benefits, lentils can be a cook's first or second best friend: they cook up quickly and work well in a variety of dishes, from soups and stews to salads and even pancakes. In fact, lentils are so popular they merit their very own annual festival in Washington State. To find out how you can celebrate the lentil, call the National Lentil Festival at 800-365-6948.

Like their fellow legumes, lentils are an ancient edible, with the Egyptians, Greeks, and Romans having enjoyed them on their dinner tables. But for many people, lentils are forever associated with the cooking of the great Indian Subcontinent, where lentils in a multitude of small lens-shaped sizes and varying colors—from red to orange to green to black—enrich mealtimes with their earthy-sweet taste. It seems that Indians even think of lentils much like Americans think of hamburgers and mac 'n' cheese: the ultimate comfort food. In restaurants, most Indian menus include one or perhaps several dals, or spiced cooked lentils.

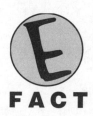

FACT

Lentils deserve special recognition, and in the United States, at least three groups focus energy on promoting this legume: The North Dakota Dry Pea and Lentil Council, the North Dakota Dry Pea and Lentil Association, and the USA Dry Pea and Lentil Council.

Working with Lentils

Most supermarkets carry the common brown lentils, but for real gastronomic explorations, you should try the tiny French green lentils and the Italian black lentils, or take a trip to an Indian grocer, whose shelves will display a variety of lentil shapes and colors. You'll find whole or split lentils, and even some lentils with the hulls removed. You might want to stock up on a lentil supply, for like their bean cousins, lentils are a bargain source of proteins and vitamins, and since they are dried, they store well for up to a year in a cool, dry place.

When it comes to the cookpot, remember that lentils require rinsing, though not generally soaking, and cook more quickly than beans; the slow-cooking French lentils and the whole black lentils need more cooking time than the other lentil varieties. Many varieties can turn mushy if overcooked, so keep an eye on them, and after about fifteen minutes of simmering, test for doneness; depending on age and variety, some lentils may require up to one hour or longer of simmering. Because of their mild flavors, lentils show up better when cooked with strong spices and onions, otherwise just enjoy them plain. For information about lentils and chickpeas, visit *www.pea-lentil.com/consumer.htm.*

Checking Out Chickpeas

Whether you call them chickpeas or garbanzo beans—or Bengal grams or Egyptian peas—these pulses are another super food, high in proteins and nutrients, low in cost. Chickpeas are also apparently good sources for molybdenum and manganese. Along with other dried pulses, garbanzos are on the USDA's recommended list for vegetables or for meat substitutes to include in your diet.

Like other legumes, chickpeas have a long past, and presumably are native to the Middle East, where their use in such ubiquitous fare as hummus and falafel make them dietary staples. But chickpeas turn up on Italian, Turkish, and Greek tables, and they have taken center stage in India—a major chickpea producer—where cooks grind up chickpeas into a flour (gram flour, or *besan*) for use in such dishes as breads, pancakes, and dumplings or use chickpeas for curries and other dishes.

Working with Chickpeas

Although purists say you have not tasted a real chickpea until you've cooked it from scratch, their preparation is somewhat time-consuming, requiring overnight soaking and lengthy simmering to tenderize them. Obviously, picking up canned chickpeas saves kitchen hassle; be sure to rinse canned chickpeas to wash away excess sodium.

Chickpeas can then make great additions to soups, salads, curries, stews, or pastas, or they can be heated and eaten solo with your choice of seasonings. You can easily even make your own hummus by puréeing chickpeas with olive oil, lemon juice, garlic, tahini paste, and some chopped parsley.

Black Bean and Plantain Burritos

SERVES 2

670 calories
23g fat
86g carbohydrates
39g protein
620mg sodium
23g fiber

These filling burritos make a luscious supper dish. But if you want to start the day with a satisfying and simple breakfast or brunch, these are good candidates. Queso fresco is a slightly salty, crumbly Mexican cheese; look for it in an Hispanic market.

1. Heat the oil in a large skillet over medium heat and add the beans, stirring and mashing them as they cook. Stir in the salsa and the seasonings and continue cooking and mashing for about 5 minutes more.

2. Split the plantain in half lengthwise and then into quarters. Spray a nonstick skillet with nonstick cooking spray and pan-fry the plantain pieces until they are browned on both sides. Remove the plantain pieces and heat the 2 tortillas in the same skillet, spraying again, as needed. When soft, place the tortillas on serving plates. Heap a portion of the beans on one side of the tortilla, place 2 pieces of plantain on the beans, and sprinkle with 2 tablespoons *queso fresco*; fold the tortilla into a burrito or taco shape. Repeat with the remaining ingredients.

INGREDIENTS:

2 tablespoons vegetable oil
2 (15.25-ounce) cans black
    beans, drained and rinsed
¼ cup salsa
1 teaspoon dried oregano
1 teaspoon ground cumin
1 teaspoon ancho chili powder
1 yellow plantain, peeled
2 (9-inch) whole wheat tortillas
4 tablespoons queso fresco, or
    other white crumbly cheese
Snipped fresh cilantro for
    garnish

What Are Plantains?

If you have not already sampled this banana look-alike—and banana variety—you'll find that plantains are so versatile that they can be eaten green in savory dishes, or allowed to ripen, even to turn black, and be used as a sweet accent in both sweet and savory fare. Popular in Latino and African countries, the plantain is a pleasing starchy fruit, but note: plantains are not eaten raw.

SERVES 6

590 calories
24g fat
65g carbohydrates
33g protein
1,800mg sodium
21g fiber

INGREDIENTS:

3 tablespoons vegetable oil
1 large onion, diced
12 ounces ground soy "meat" crumbles
1 tablespoon chili powder, or more to taste
1 (15-ounce) can golden hominy
1 (15½-ounce) can canary beans, drained and rinsed
1 (15½-ounce) can pigeon peas, drained and rinsed
1 cup green salsa
1 cup Mexican beer, or more as needed
Salt and freshly ground black pepper to taste
3 tomatillos, chopped, for garnish
Grated cheese for garnish
Chopped fresh cilantro for garnish
Diced avocados for garnish
Toasted pumpkin seeds for garnish

Golden West Chili

This chili, which is as bright and sunny as a day in California, can be altered to suit your taste. Just keep the proportions about the same. Serve this with fresh flour tortillas.

1. Heat the oil in a large saucepan over medium heat and sauté the onion until partially golden, about 5 minutes. Add the soy "meat" crumbles and continue cooking for 3 or 4 more minutes. Stir in the chili powder. Add the hominy, beans, pigeon peas, salsa, and beer and stir well.

2. Reduce the heat to medium-low and continue cooking and stirring about 8 minutes more. Season with salt and pepper. Serve in individual bowls, garnishing as desired.

What Is Hominy?

If you are not from the South nor have ever eaten that Mexican classic *posole*, you may not be familiar with the white corn kernel known as hominy. Made from dried corn kernels that have been treated chemically, hominy has a pleasant texture and mild taste. In the Southwest and in Mexico, larger-kernel hominy is available and is known as posole. The smaller hominy is sold canned in most supermarkets; look for the larger variety at a Latino market.

Mediterranean Stew

*Serve this stew, redolent with the flavors of the sunny
Mediterranean, with warmed pita bread.*

1. Heat the olive oil in a large saucepan over medium heat and sauté
   the garlic for 2 to 3 minutes or until golden.

2. Reduce the heat to medium-low. Stir in the chickpeas, cannellini
   beans, roasted tomatoes, artichoke hearts, broth, Parmesan cheese,
   crushed red pepper, oregano, salt, and pepper. Cook and stir for
   about 10 minutes. Serve in individual bowls, garnishing as desired.

SERVES 4

390 calories
13g fat
52g carbohydrates
15g protein
1,180mg sodium
9g fiber

INGREDIENTS:

3 tablespoons olive oil

3 cloves garlic, crushed and
   minced

1 (15½-ounce) can chickpeas,
   drained and rinsed

1 (19-ounce) can cannellini
   beans, drained and rinsed

2 cups roasted tomatoes

1½ cups artichoke hearts,
   quartered

1 cup vegetable broth

4 tablespoons grated Parmesan
   cheese

1 teaspoon crushed red pepper,
   or to taste

1 teaspoon dried oregano

Salt and freshly ground black
   pepper to taste

Chopped sun-dried tomatoes for
   garnish

Chopped Italian parsley for
   garnish

Garlic-seasoned croutons for
   garnish

Crumbled feta cheese for
   garnish

Fresh oregano leaves for garnish

Fava Bean Hummus with Kalamata Olives and Pistachios

SERVES 6

240 calories
17g fat
18g carbohydrates
8g protein
150mg sodium
5g fiber

INGREDIENTS:

1 (15-ounce) can fava beans, drained and rinsed
3 cloves garlic, or to taste
Juice from 1 lemon, or more to taste
3 tablespoons olive oil, or more as needed to process
1 to 2 tablespoons tahini paste
Salt and freshly ground black pepper to taste
½ cup minced parsley
¾ cup toasted pistachios

If you need extra liquid to help purée the fava beans, you may add olive oil or a splash of vegetable broth, but don't overdo it. The hummus should be thick, not runny. You may serve this with toasted pita pieces or bagel chips or with fresh vegetables for dunking.

1. Put the beans, garlic, lemon juice, olive oil, tahini, salt, and pepper into a food processor or blender and purée.

2. Spoon the mixture into a bowl and stir in the parsley and pistachios. Chill until serving time.

What Is Tahini?

This Middle Eastern condiment is a paste made from a blending of toasted sesame seeds and vegetable oil. Tahini is used in numerous Middle Eastern dishes and is essential in the making of hummus. It is readily available in well-stocked supermarkets.

Connie's Delicious Refried Beans

Although canned refried beans are convenient, starting from scratch yields a spectacular flavor absent in the canned version. This Americanized take on refried beans packs a wonderful punch, and it is a dish you'll want to make often, especially if you like burritos, tacos, and quesadillas. These also are terrific for breakfast topped with eggs poached in a thick salsa.

1. Soak the rinsed beans overnight in cold water to cover by 2 inches. Drain them well and rinse the beans again.

2. Put the beans and the onion in a large saucepan with about 8 cups water, or to cover by 2 inches. Bring the water to a boil and reduce the heat to medium-low; skim off any scum. Stir in the chili seasonings, the cumin seeds, and the jalapeño. Cook, checking on the water level and stirring occasionally, for 3 to 4 hours or until the beans are tender and the water is almost absorbed. Add the salsa and salt.

3. Heat the vegetable oil in a large skillet and, by spoonfuls, put the beans in the skillet and, using a potato masher of the back of a large spoon, mash and fry them until the beans are relatively smooth, repeating until all the beans are mashed and fried.

SERVES 6

320 calories
6g fat
51g carbohydrates
18g protein
95mg sodium
15g fiber

INGREDIENTS:

1 (1 pound bag) dried pinto beans, rinsed and picked clean

1 cup chopped onion, or more if desired

1 package dried hot chili seasoning

1 package dried mild chili seasoning

1 tablespoon roasted cumin seeds, pounded with a mortar and pestle

1 jalapeño chile, seeded and diced

Salsa to taste

Salt to taste

2 tablespoons vegetable oil, or more as needed

SERVES 4

280 calories
13g fat
31g carbohydrates
12g protein
420mg sodium
11g fiber

INGREDIENTS:

3 tablespoons olive oil
1 large sweet onion, thinly
  sliced
5 cloves garlic, minced
2 cups cooked lentils
3 tomatoes, quartered
2 banana peppers, stemmed and
  quartered lengthwise
2 Italian-style soy "sausages,"
  thinly sliced
1 portobello mushroom, thinly
  sliced
½ to 1 cup vegetable broth, or
  more as needed
Salt and freshly ground black
  pepper to taste

Lentils cook up fast, but if you are in a big hurry, use canned lentils for convenience's sake. Offer this stew with slices of hot, buttery baguette, which you can spark with sprinkles of garlic powder, and serve a simple salad of lightly dressed greens.

1. Heat the oil in a large skillet over medium heat and sauté the onion for 8 to 10 minutes or until golden. Add the garlic, lentils, tomatoes, peppers, "sausages," and mushroom, stirring well.

2. Reduce the heat to medium-low and continue cooking until the onions and peppers soften, about 10 minutes. Add the vegetable broth as the mixture begins to dry out. Stir in the salt and pepper. Serve hot.

Sprout Sandwich with Avocado

This simple bagel treat works well at any time of day. It's easy to double or triple this recipe for others in the family.

Slice the bagel in half widthwise and toast it. Mix the remaining ingredients together and spread on both halves of the bagel. Serve.

SERVES 1

700 calories
40g fat
76g carbohydrates
16g protein
880mg sodium
18g fiber

INGREDIENTS:

1 whole wheat bagel, toasted
½ ripe avocado, diced
4 tablespoons mixed sprouts
2 tablespoons mayonnaise, or more as desired
2 tablespoons toasted pumpkin seeds
1 teaspoon Dijon mustard
Salt and freshly ground black pepper to taste

SERVES 2

600 calories
20g fat
92g carbohydrates
16g protein
700mg sodium
14g fiber

INGREDIENTS:
2 tablespoons vegetable oil
1 onion, diced
1 tomato, diced
*2 tablespoons minced fresh
    ginger*
1 tablespoon minced garlic
1 teaspoon ground turmeric
*1 (15¼-ounce) can chickpeas,
    drained and rinsed*
*1 teaspoon curry powder, or
    more to taste*
1 teaspoon ground cumin
*½ bunch fresh cilantro, coarsely
    chopped*
Salt to taste
*½ cup plain nonfat or whole
    milk yogurt*
*½ cup sweet or hot chutney, or
    to taste*

Fried Chickpeas with Yogurt

*A flavorful Indian favorite spiked with chutney, this entrée
comes together in minutes and is a perfect accompaniment to
cooked basmati rice and hot, fresh naan, the popular Indian
bread.*

1. Heat the oil in a large skillet over medium heat and sauté the onion
    and tomato until the vegetables soften. Add the ginger, garlic, and
    turmeric and cook 2 to 3 minutes more or until the flavors are com-
    bined.

2. Add the chickpeas, curry powder, and cumin and cook, stirring
    often, for about 5 minutes. Add the cilantro and salt, stirring well.
    Stir in the yogurt and cook 2 minutes more. Serve with a dollop of
    chutney on each portion.

White Bean Soup with Chipotle Croutons

If you can find it, be sure to use the chorizo in this soup. It's tube shaped and packed in plastic; unwrap the "sausage" and sauté the crumbles until golden. Sprinkle them into the soup once it's hot. A splash of heavy cream turns this soup into a lush treat.

1. Put 1 can of beans into the blender or food processor. Add the tomatoes, oregano, chipotle sauce, salt and pepper, and 2 tablespoons olive oil and process until fairly smooth. Pour into a saucepan.

2. If using the chorizo, heat 2 more tablespoons olive oil in a skillet over medium-low heat and crumble and sauté the sausage.

3. Heat the soup in a saucepan over medium heat, stirring in the remaining beans and the chorizo "sausage" if using. To serve, ladle soup into individual bowls and garnish with the croutons, red onions, and cilantro.

What Is Chipotle?

The chipotle is the smoked and dried ripe jalapeño chile pepper that has turned red on the vine. Chipotles are readily available packed in a smoky-hot sauce in cans. Using the whole chile pepper or some of the sauce perks up any flavor.

SERVES 4

730 calories
38g fat
71g carbohydrates
24g protein
1,680mg sodium
11g fiber

INGREDIENTS:

2 (15½-ounce) cans navy or other white beans, drained and rinsed
1½ cups fresh or canned tomatoes
1 teaspoon dried oregano
1 teaspoon chipotle sauce
Salt and freshly ground black pepper to taste
2 tablespoons olive oil, or 4 tablespoons if using chorizo
1 (12-ounce) package soy chorizo "sausage," optional
1 cup garlic croutons sprinkled with ground chipotle chiles
2 tablespoons diced red onion
Chopped fresh cilantro for garnish

SERVES 8

510 calories
29g fat
57g carbohydrates
9g protein
670mg sodium
2g fiber

INGREDIENTS:
½ cup crunchy peanut butter
1 (8-ounce) package soy cream
    cheese, at room temperature
¾ cup packed brown sugar
1 large egg, lightly beaten
3 tablespoons cornstarch
½ cup chocolate morsels
1 (16.3-ounce) tube flaky
    refrigerator biscuits

Peanut Butter Cups

A baked takeoff on a popular candy, these biscuits make a delicious dessert, but why not serve them for breakfast as well? Or even pop one into a lunch box. Use 3½-inch-round muffin tins.

1. Preheat the oven to 375°F. Spray the tins with nonstick cooking spray.

2. Combine the peanut butter, cream cheese, and sugar in a mixing bowl and beat until smooth. Add the egg and cornstarch and beat again. Fold the morsels in by hand.

3. Roll out the biscuits one at a time on a lightly floured surface and fit each into a muffin cup so that it forms a "crust." Spoon the peanut butter mixture into each biscuit crust. Reduce the temperature to 350°F.

4. Bake the muffins for 25 to 30 minutes, or until the center feels firm to the touch. Remove from the oven and cool to firm completely.

CHAPTER 9

Side and Entrée Salads

In this health-conscious twenty-first century, people regard a salad as more than just a refresher: it's often the entire meal, composed of an exquisite array of ingredients that provide color, flavor, texture, nutrients, and, often, pleasure. For the vegetarian looking to vary the menu, a salad provides a tempting option.

9

All about Salads

If you think about it, the salad has finally come into its own: no longer a last-minute bowl of greens or a composition of canned fruits or vegetables, the salad has its own hardware: the salad bowl, the salad tongs, lettuce spinners, choppers, and special salad dressing dispensers, to name a few items. And it even takes center stage at most supermarkets, where salad bars display a wide range of greens and salad extras. Indeed, the salad should often be a main player in vegetarian meals. Winifred Gibbs, in the 1912 *Economical Cooking* cookbook, advised her readers, "As a matter of fact, a salad should be an ordinary dish served as often as possible rather than an uncommon one."

History of Salads

Food historians tell us that ancient Greeks and Romans enjoyed a bowl of mixed greens at mealtimes, lightly dressing them with oil, vinegar, and salt—hence, the word *salad*, a derivative of the Latin word for salt, *sal*. But apparently the salad's history actually stems from a time thousands of years further back, when greens as salads graced dinner tables in the Mediterranean region long before Roman times.

While salads may have slipped into obscurity for several centuries during the Dark Ages and beyond, these bowls of greens once again became mealtime favorites when the Renaissance age began in the fourteenth century. By then, European cooks had learned to fill out the salad bowl with other ingredients, from eggs to cooked vegetables, and much more. Of course, the salad took on other forms as well: the Dutch refined the coleslaw concept; Germans delighted in warm dressed potatoes; the Tuscans elevated the bread salad, the *panzanella*, into a tomato delight with tomatoes and sliced or cubed bread; and early Americans heaped fruits together in a bowl and called the result "ambrosia" and later, "fruit cocktail."

Fast forward to the mid-twentieth century, when salads took steps forward in the American menu. By that time, the chef's salad, originated probably by chef Louis Diat at the Ritz-Carlton Hotel in New York City, had its imitators. The much-loved Cobb salad likely hails from Hollywood's Brown Derby restaurant, where its original owner, Mr. Robert Cobb, reputedly whipped it up from leftovers ones night. The ubiquitous Caesar Salad, probably created by Italian-born Caesare Cardini in his Tijuana, Mexico, restaurant in the 1920s, launched itself onto the public's most-loved salad list. Today, you can scarcely find an American restaurant without a chef's take on the Caesar salad.

At the end of the twentieth and on into the twenty-first centuries, salads have become designer creations, often on upscale restaurant menus as compellingly beautiful as the main course itself. The inventive chef turns to a wide-ranging palate of colors and a broad spectrum of textures to turn the once-simple bowl of crisp greens into a fanciful dish. But despite all the frills, lettuce generally remains the salad bowl basic.

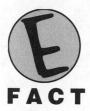

FACT

Strange salads—or at least what modern cooks might question—have made their way to the table, such as a 1920s American salad of cottage cheese flavored with ketchup, rolled into balls and served on watercress; and from New Zealand in decades past, the salad of cream cheese rolled in grated carrots.

Let Us Eat Lettuce

For the modern-day shopper, the array of true lettuce varieties in the produce section and at farmers' markets has exploded, from the time-honored iceberg heads and romaine, to Bibb, Boston, Ruby (or red leaf), chicory, corn salad, oak leaf, Buttercrunch, and Black Seeded Simpson, plus dozens and dozens more. According to the CDC, all these varieties fall into one of the four main categories: crisphead, butterhead, looseleaf, and cos or romaine.

Healthful Lettuces

Probably most people think of lettuce as nothing more than a bland conveyance of dressing flavors or the background for other, more interesting ingredients. But the fact is that most lettuce leaves, while not nutrient powerhouses, do convey some essential vitamins and that all-important fiber all people need. Besides, for folks on a diet, few foods contain fewer calories, ounce for ounce, and lettuce has no fat or cholesterol. For example, one cup of chopped raw romaine lettuce contains ten calories and zero grams of fat, cholesterol, and sodium. Both the calories and fat come with what you put into the salad bowl to keep the lettuce company.

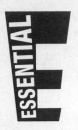

Fortunately for the avid gardener, most lettuce varieties flourish in garden plots and containers for cool- to warm-weather enjoyment, making life simple for those who want ultrafresh greens for the salad bowl. For lettuce-growing inspiration, visit *www.urbanext.uiuc.edu/veggies/lettuce1 .html*.

Experts point out the lettuce leaves—particularly those that are darker green—do contain such vitamins as A and C, and offer calcium, potassium, and beta-carotene. Plus lettuce leaves are a good source for those all-important phytonutrients that work as antioxidants to fight illness. Even the iceberg lettuce, so often spurned by salad enthusiasts as being a tasteless second-best, not only has made a glamorous salad-bowl comeback, but it also contains some vitamin A. Note that nutrient values also vary by lettuce type.

Caring for Lettuces

Because they are tender, salad greens require careful handling, from garden plot or market to the table; even the compact iceberg head, which seems almost indestructible, needs careful tending at home. When making your lettuce selection, pick those heads that have crisp leaves with no signs of wilting or decay. As soon as you get your lettuce home, the CDC recommends immediately wrapping the greens in plastic and refrigerating them. Some cooks prefer to rinse the leaves in cold water first, dry them thoroughly, and then wrap them in paper towels and place in a perforated plastic bag before refrigerating them. Remember, wet leaves spoil very quickly, even when refrigerated.

Whichever your preference, all salad greens need thorough rinsing in cold water before use; never use soap on lettuce leaves. Rinsing in several changes of water removes grit, any insects, and any other possible contaminants. The best way to dry off leaves is with a salad spinner, which twirls away excess moisture, leaving you with leaves ready for the salad bowl. Otherwise, you can gingerly shake leaves in several layers of absorbent kitchen towels.

When assembling your salad—whether it is a simple toss of dressed greens or a more elaborately composed entrée salad—let the greens go in last, making sure to trim away and discard any wilted or discolored leaves. And dress your salad just before serving to preserve the greens' crisp texture.

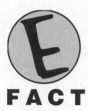

FACT

According to 2005 figures cited by the USDA's Economic Research Service, and published in the *Los Angeles Daily News* in 2007, Americans consumed about thirty-four and a half pounds of lettuce per person; twenty-two pounds of this total reflected consumption of iceberg lettuce.

Building a Tasty Salad

Building an exciting salad means thinking outside the bowl. What would work well? To figure out what you want to toss into the mix, stroll the produce aisles, and get creative. Salads can contain almost any ingredient and can become an international dish by varying flavors and textures.

Other Salad Greens and Colors

When creating your salad, make it interesting by combining several lettuce varieties—this adds color and texture to your bowl. You might also want to include other nonlettuce greens, such as endive, sorrel, spinach, watercress, arugula, fennel, and radicchio, as well as parsley and a host of vegetables such as sprouts, radishes, and celery.

And what about flowers? Ever had marigolds, nasturtiums, pansies, or rose petals for true flavor and visual excitement? Of course, with flowers, you must be certain to use only edible ones and nonsprayed petals.

One exciting addition to the lettuce aisle is the packaging of greens called mesclun, which really means a mix of young salad greens. Apparently, this idea originated in France, where cooks wanted to serve salads with a variety of tastes and textures. The typical mesclun mix may contain chervil, chicory, dandelion, and mustard greens, and additionally, spinach, radicchio, and kale.

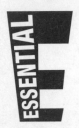

Cooking with flowers has a long kitchen pedigree; food historians point out that early Romans, Chinese, and Indians had favorite blooms for their culinary creations. Americans, too, have enjoyed flowers in their recipes. In an 1891 newspaper recipe article, M. Sherwood suggested using bright nasturtium blossoms in a buttercup lettuce salad. Want to try your hand at cooking with flowers? Check out *www.beyondblossoms .com/blog/2006/05/08/cooking-with-flowers*.

The newest salad superstars are the microgreens, which are really some of the same greens varieties sold as mesclun, but microgreens are cut and harvested when much smaller plants, perhaps only one to two inches high. Restaurant chefs delight in garnishing fancy dishes with a handful of microgreens, but as of this writing these greens are not readily available for the consumer, except at some farmers' markets.

Using Cooked Vegetables

You can definitely expand the boundaries of your salad fixings by selecting colorful vegetables, such as beets, carrots, snow peas, broccoli, peas, asparagus, and green beans—to name just a few. Ready them for the salad bowl by trimming and blanching. Even leftover veggies can add an unexpected texture to the salad bowl.

Cooked or canned beans are obvious salad choices as well, and here you have so many alternatives in the supermarket that you can turn the whole salad bowl into a mix of beans, using greens as a garnish and onions or other vegetables for crunch.

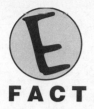

FACT

Using roasted peppers in the salad bowl adds both color and a certain drama. Select a very firm, ripe sweet bell pepper and rub it all over in olive oil. Put it on a baking sheet, and broil it, turning it often, until the pepper's skin is charred on all sides. Remove the pepper from the broiler, and place it in a paper bag or in a heatproof bowl covered with plastic wrap or foil. When cool enough to handle, slice off the stem end, and rub off the charred skin. Discard the seeds and ribs. Preserve it in olive oil until ready to use. Do not run the pepper (or peppers, as you can do several at a time) under water as this washes away their flavorful juices.

Potato Salads and More

Thanks to a surge in consumer interest, many markets now stock a range of potatoes in varying sizes, shapes, and colors. But not every variety is destined for the salad bowl. Best for cutting and dicing are the waxy potatoes, such as the red-skinned, low-starch varieties, because they hold their shape well. To make the correct potato selections, go to this website: *www.potatoes.com/VarietiesAndUses.cfm*.

Grains and Pastas

Both grains and pastas provide a mild flavor profile for salad greens and vegetables, but they also add texture, color, and nutrients. Of the grains used in a salad, perhaps the most famous is the wheat that goes into the Middle Eastern tabbouleh, or bulgur salad, made with abundant parsley and an olive oil dressing. For salads, select grains that stay intact after cooking and don't turn to mush, especially after you dress the grains.

As for pastas, consider both the Western and Asian pastas, which can add a subtle taste and texture to your salad bowl. Italian pastas come in so many different shapes—and some colors—that they can provide a visual feast. But you must take care to cook them properly so that they don't clump together after cooking. Asian rice, buckwheat, and wheat noodles, while not formed into appealing shapes, still offer a different flavor and texture background: thin rice noodles, for example, can be crisped with deep-frying or made into tender lengths after boiling and draining.

Add-Ons

As you look at your salad bowl, you worry that something is missing. Do you want to add something quirky like scallion brushes, rose petals, or cut-up fruit? Emphasize flavors with a sprinkling of fresh herbs? What about softening the crunch of grains with avocado cubes? Enriching the salad with shredded cheese? Or adding texture to soft lettuces with a toss-in of seeds, nuts, or croutons? As you can see, what you add to the salad bowl is really limited only by your imagination—and common sense.

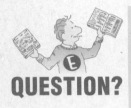

QUESTION?

How do I make my own croutons?
For homemade croutons: Select a textured sourdough bread—or other textured loaf—trim off the crusts (or leave them on for more texture) and slice the loaf into ½- to 1-inch cubes. Toast them in a skillet with 3 to 4 tablespoons olive oil over medium heat, reduce the heat to medium-low, and continue cooking and turning them until the cubes are browned on all sides. You can heighten their flavor by add crushed garlic to the oil. And when the cubes are browned, toss them in a bowl with grated Parmesan cheese, if you wish.

The Final Touch: Dressings

The final salad element is the dressing, and to assemble that you have at hand assorted oils, vinegars, seasonings, and enrichments such as mayonnaise, cream, sour cream, and yogurt. Unless you want the dressing to play the leading role—such as in the Caesar salad, whose dressing really defines the recipe—you should carefully judge which elements to select.

Choice of Oils

Classical cooks turn to rich, dark-green extra-virgin olive oils for their dressing basics, but these oils have a pronounced fruity flavor that may overpower other salad ingredients. Other strong oils include walnut oil, hazelnut oil, and, especially, toasted sesame oil, which you would use only as an accent, not a major ingredient.

Milder flavored oils good for salad dressing include canola oil, corn oil, safflower oil, and sunflower oil. Whichever you select—and you should try out several types to find one you like—be sure your oil has not been made from genetically modified (GMO) seeds. Note that olive oil in particular is considered a heart-healthy oil because it is high in mono- and polyunsaturated fats.

Choice of Vinegars

As with oil selections, regular, sherry and wine, rice, balsamic, and herb- or berry-infused vinegars make salad seasoning more like an art project than a culinary one. As with oil choices, keep in mind the end result. You would not want to use a harsh white vinegar, for example, if dressing a sweetish fruit salad. And for the most delicate salads, you could simply use a squeeze of fresh citrus juice with a drizzle of oil.

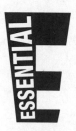

You can quickly make a basic and foolproof vinaigrette by following a simple oil-to-vinegar ratio: one part vinegar to three to four parts olive oil. Then you add salt and pepper to taste, and to make this dressing fancier, diced shallots, and a dash of Dijon mustard. Once you have perfected the basic dressing, get creative.

Choice of Seasonings

You might consider a few flavor enhancers, such as crushed garlic or chopped fresh herbs, maybe a touch of mayonnaise for a creamier dressing, minced shallots, perhaps even minced ginger for a fruit dish. A careful selection of these background seasonings can really amplify the dressing and turn a simple greens dish into a memorable one.

570 calories
21g fat
87g carbohydrates
11g protein
790mg sodium
3g fiber

INGREDIENTS:
3 cups cooked rice
1 cup cashews
1 cup canned lychees, drained
½ cup wasabi-flavored peas
½ cup candied ginger cubes
3 tablespoons soy sauce
1 tablespoon vegetable oil
1 teaspoon toasted sesame oil
Rice seasoning to taste

Warm Rice Salad

Let the rice cool to room temperature, or just slightly warmer, before assembling this salad; this is not meant to be a hot dish.

1. Combine the rice, cashews, lychees, peas, and ginger in a large salad bowl.

2. In a small bowl, combine the soy sauce, vegetable oil, and sesame oil and mix well.

3. Dress the salad with this mixture, tossing well. Sprinkle with the rice seasoning and serve.

What Is Rice Seasoning?
A Japanese dry condiment used for perking up rice and other dishes, rice seasoning is available at Asian markets and well-stocked supermarkets. Check the label before you buy; some brands contains dried shrimp or shaved bonito flakes. The basic ingredients are crumbled seaweed, sesame seeds, salt, and sugar. You just shake out what you want from the small jar.

Asian Fusion Salad

This Asian fusion greens salad uses Thai and Chinese ingredients tossed with Western baby spinach and olive oil for a pleasing result. Note that although the Thai chili sauce is slightly sweet, it also provides a chili kick.

1. Combine the coconut milk, Thai chili sauce, soy sauce, and olive oil, mix well, and set aside.

2. Combine the spinach, watercress, and water chestnuts in a salad bowl, add the dressing, and toss until the leaves are well coated. Sprinkle the crushed rice crackers and cashews over top, toss again, and serve.

SERVES 2 AS AN ENTRÉE, 4 TO 6 AS A SIDE SALAD

440 calories
27g fat
42g carbohydrates
11g protein
1400mg sodium
6g fiber

INGREDIENTS:
3 tablespoons lite coconut milk
3 tablespoons Thai chili sauce
2 tablespoons soy sauce
1 tablespoon olive oil
2 cups baby spinach
1 bunch watercress, trimmed
1 (8-ounce) can sliced water chestnuts
8 sesame-flavored rice crackers, crumbled
½ cup crushed cashews
1 bunch watercress, rinsed and trimmed into 1-inch length

Asian Chopped Salad with Crispy Noodles and Kim Chee

SERVES 4

560 calories
26g fat
59g carbohydrates
25g protein
920mg sodium
9g fiber

INGREDIENTS:

2 bunches scallions, trimmed and thinly sliced

8 ounces Thai-flavored baked tofu, diced

2 cups baby spinach

1 cup cubed water chestnuts

1 cup crumbled crispy chow mein noodles

1 cup fresh shelled edamame

½ cup kim chee, drained and chopped

½ cup chopped baby corn

2 tablespoons toasted sesame seeds

Asian-style commercial salad dressing to taste

Kim chee is the peppery condiment that is the staple of the Korean table. Made from pickled and fermented cabbage and/ or other vegetables and other assorted add-ins, kim chee is available at well-stocked supermarkets in the refrigerated case of the produce section. Otherwise, search out a local Korean or pan-Asian market.

Combine all the ingredients in a salad bowl and toss with the dressing. Serve.

What Are Chow Mein Noodles and Baby Corn?

Most markets stock noodles, or chow mein noodles, that are already deep-fried until crispy. These add a zesty crunch to any salad mixture but particularly to one that is Asian inspired. Some markets also stock deep-fried rice noodles for a change in pace. The baby corn that often turns up in Chinese stir-fries is corn that is harvested early just after the silk is produced; however, you can find seeds for baby corn variety on the web. The tiny cobs retain crispiness while adding a sweet undertone to other dishes. These are readily available canned.

Mediterranean Potato Salad

Take advantage of the many different sizes of potatoes stocked in major supermarkets and at farmers' markets. You will probably find the fingerlings in assorted colors, as well as potatoes as small as a thimble and others tinged purple or blue. Mix and match, for the most interesting potato salad.

1. Cut the potatoes up until they are of a uniform size. Put them into a salad bowl and add the scallions, grape tomatoes, eggs, parsley, olives, and "bacon" bits.

2. Mix together the mayonnaise, buttermilk, olive oil, smoked paprika, salt, and pepper. Whisk together until well mixed. Dress the salad, tossing gently to coat all the ingredients. Serve.

SERVES 4

400 calories
16g fat
54g carbohydrates
11g protein
430mg sodium
7g fiber

INGREDIENTS:

2 pounds assorted potatoes, cooked and cooled
1 bunch scallions, thinly sliced
1 cup grape tomatoes
2 hard-boiled eggs, quartered
1 cup chopped Italian flat-leaf parsley
¾ cup pitted Niçoise olives
3 tablespoons soy "bacon" bits
2 tablespoons mayonnaise
2 tablespoons buttermilk
1 tablespoon olive oil
1 teaspoon smoked paprika
Salt and freshly ground black pepper to taste

SERVES 4

180 calories
15g fat
13g carbohydrates
3g protein
10mg sodium
8g fiber

INGREDIENTS:

*2 large ripe avocados, coarsely
    chopped
1 small white onion, diced
1 tomato, unpeeled and diced
1 jalapeño chile, thinly sliced
Juice of 1 lime
Salt to taste*

Maria's Guacamole

*Plan to make this soon before you eat it, as avocados tend to
discolor quickly unless tightly wrapped and chilled with their
pits.*

Gently combine all the ingredients in a serving bowl and pass as a
salad or appetizer.

What Is Guacamole?

Food historians suggest that guacamole, that beloved salad or dip made
from avocados, was a favored Aztec food. It certainly has staying power,
for it's so popular today that manufacturers have figured out ways to
package it for mass marketing. Because avocados darken easily when
exposed to air, save any leftovers with the pits and keep in a tightly sealed
container in the refrigerator.

Crispy Chinese Cabbage with Shredded Peanut "Chicken"

You might want to accompany this salad with crispy spring rolls and a peanut dipping sauce. For variety's sake, try using crispy tofu in place of the "chicken" strips.

1. Put the cabbage shreds, julienned pepper, peanuts, and cilantro leaves in a large bowl. Set aside.

2. Heat 1 tablespoon oil in a large wok or skillet over medium heat and stir-fry the "chicken" strips and bamboo shoots for 1 minute. Set aside.

3. Mix the ¼ cup oil, peanut butter, soy sauce, garlic, vinegar, sugar, and crushed red pepper, whisking together to mix well. Blend the dressing ingredients with a whisk until smooth in a small bowl and set aside.

4. Add the "chicken" strips and bamboo shoots to the cabbage mixture and toss with the salad dressing to coat the ingredients well. Serve.

SERVES 4 TO 6

410 calories
29g fat
24g carbohydrates
21g protein
750mg sodium
7g fiber

INGREDIENTS:

5 cups shredded napa cabbage (about 1¼ pounds)
1 sweet red pepper, seeded and julienned
1 cup roasted peanuts
¾ cup fresh cilantro leaves
1 tablespoon plus ¼ cup vegetable oil
2 (6-ounce) packages soy "chicken" strips
1 cup shredded bamboo shoots, rinsed and drained
3 tablespoons crunchy peanut butter
3 tablespoons soy sauce
3 cloves garlic, minced
3 tablespoons rice vinegar
3 tablespoons sugar
1 to 2 teaspoons crushed red pepper

SERVES 4 TO 6

For 1 tablespoon dressing:
35 calories
3g fat
2g carbohydrates
0g protein
125mg sodium
0g fiber

For salad:
330 calories
21g fat
19g carbohydrates
16g protein
1,040mg sodium
7g fiber

INGREDIENTS:
Dressing
¼ cup soy sauce
¼ cup vegetable oil
3 tablespoons sesame oil
Zest of 1 orange, finely grated
Juice of 1 orange
2 tablespoons sugar or to taste
1 to 2 teaspoons crushed red pepper
2 teaspoons minced fresh ginger

Salad
2 tablespoons vegetable oil
¼ pound snow peas
2 (6-ounce) packages soy "steak" strips
2 cups bok choy leaves, torn into pieces
4 to 6 mustard green leaves, torn into pieces
1 bunch scallions, trimmed and cut into 1-inch pieces
1 cup crumbled chow mein noodles
3 to 4 red chiles sliced on the diagonal for garnish
Fresh cilantro leaves for garnish

Orange "Beef" on Greens with Crispy Noodles

Snow peas, slivered green onions, and sturdy bok choy provide the backdrop for this robust salad, which could become a fixture at your table. For convenience's sake, you could substitute the commercial grated orange rind for fresh orange zest, but you will not achieve the same lively citrus flavor. Store any remaining dressing in the refrigerator.

1. Combine the dressing ingredients in a small bowl, stirring well to dissolve the sugar. Set aside.

2. Heat a wok or large skillet over medium-high heat and when the pan is hot, add 1 tablespoon oil. When the oil is hot, stir-fry the snow peas for 30 seconds, drizzling 1 teaspoon dressing over the vegetables while stirring. Transfer the vegetables to a salad bowl. Add the remaining 1 tablespoon oil to the wok and when hot, stir-fry the "steak" strips for 30 seconds; add 1 tablespoon dressing and stir-fry 30 seconds more. Transfer the "steak" strips to the bowl.

3. Toss the bok choy and mustard green leaves together with the snow peas, scallions, and "beef" strips and add the chow mein noodles. Add enough dressing to coat the leaves, tossing the greens to mix well. Garnish the salad with the red chiles and cilantro and serve.

Best Tuscan Bread and Heirloom Tomato Salad

SERVES 4

360 calories
26g fat
27g carbohydrates
6g protein
990mg sodium
5g fiber

Inspired by the traditional Tuscan panzanella (bread salad), this summer special showcases the heirloom tomato in its many different colors and sizes, so be sure to select several different varieties. It's so colorful and delicious that you may end up eating it every day during tomato season. Trouble is, the tomatoes lose their glamour when chilled, so eat and make it at one sitting—if possible.

1. Combine the tomatoes, bread cubes, olives, pepperoncini, feta cheese, and basil leaves in a large salad or mixing bowl.

2. Mix together the olive oil, vinegar, garlic, salt, and pepper, stirring well. Pour over the tomato mixture, tossing to combine.

3. Set aside for 15 minutes so the bread can absorb the dressing before serving.

INGREDIENTS:

About 2 pounds heirloom
   tomatoes, cubed
3 cups bread cubes
1 cup pitted kalamata olives or
   ½ cup pitted Niçoise olives
½ cup sliced pepperoncini
⅓ cup crumbled feta cheese
¼ cup julienned fresh basil
   leaves
⅓ cup extra-virgin olive oil, or
   more as needed
3 tablespoons red wine vinegar
1 tablespoon minced garlic, or
   to taste
Salt and freshly ground black
   pepper to taste

SERVES 4

280 calories
8g fat
33g carbohydrates
20g protein
860mg sodium
7g fiber

INGREDIENTS:

*About 6 cups fresh baby
    spinach, well rinsed and
    dried*
3 hard-boiled eggs, quartered
*1 (15½-ounce) can navy beans,
    drained and rinsed*
½ to 1 red onion, diced
½ cup soy "bacon" bits
½ cup toasted pumpkin seeds
1 to 2 jalapeños, thinly sliced
*Commercial salad dressing, as
    desired*

Spinach Salad

*You'll find dozens of recipes for spinach salads, but this
particular dish has some unexpected flavors. A rich Thousand
Island dressing mixed with salsa to taste accents the flavors
well. Leftovers are great.*

Combine the spinach, eggs, beans, onion, "bacon" bits, pumpkin
seeds, and jalapeños in the salad bowl. Dress as desired and serve.

Orange Salad

A healthful salad that makes a visual impact.

1. Combine the squash, carrots, and papaya in a large salad bowl. Set aside.

2. Stir together the ginger, lime juice, yogurt, honey, olive oil, salt, and pepper until well combined. Toss the dressing with the salad ingredients and serve.

SERVES 4

160 calories
4g fat
32g carbohydrates
3g protein
40mg sodium
7g fiber

INGREDIENTS:

3 cups cubed butternut squash, drizzled with olive oil and roasted
2 carrots, shredded
2 cups diced papaya
2 tablespoons shredded fresh ginger
Juice of 1 lime
2 tablespoons plain yogurt
1 tablespoon honey, or to taste
1 tablespoon olive oil
Salt and freshly ground black pepper

CHAPTER 10

Soy's Celebrity

Soy in all its many guises has gotten big press. Touted as an amazing food, a terrific protein source, and a cholesterol-free ingredient, soy wins recognition as a staple of the vegetarian diet. Its culinary benefits deserve merit, too, for when turned into bland tofu, fermented tempeh, soymilk and soy dairy-free alternatives, flour, and the various meat analogs, soy works well in many different recipes.

What Is Soy?

A legume native to China, the soybean has a cultivation history that dates back to the earliest eras of Chinese civilization—and, many believe, the ancient Chinese considered the soybean as one of the five sacred grains, joining with rice, two forms of millet, and wheat.

In the intervening centuries, food alchemists discovered the merits of the little soybean and realized that when processed in one or another way—fermenting, coagulating its liquid, or grinding the dried bean into flour—or eaten whole, the bean had great protein and seasoning potentials. Indeed, it's hard to imagine Chinese and other Asian foods prepared without the requisite flavor boost from soy sauce.

It's unclear how much bean curd, or tofu, the average Chinese eats today. If you take into account the published results of Dr. T. Colin Campbell's long-term project on China's health and diet, known as the China Study, soy seemingly is eaten only as a condiment, at least in certain parts of China. Thus it provides only a fraction of the Chinese protein intake.

This seems to contradict the prevalence of soy-based dishes in China and Taiwan. Indeed, Chinese Buddhists in their vegetarian menus have relied on soy—and other vegetables—to help create and structure their cuisine. As a health commentary, Campbell has also noted that those who ate the most legumes, basically soybeans, had lower blood cholesterol levels.

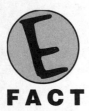

FACT

Did you know that there is a special April celebration that focuses on soyfoods? According to the Soyfoods Council, April is National Soyfoods Month, a celebration proclaimed in 1998 by the Soyfoods Association of North America.

Elsewhere in Asia, soy in many different forms is an ingredient to some degree in the diets of Malaysians, Filipinos, Thais, Vietnamese, Burmese, Koreans, and Indonesians. But perhaps throughout Asian countries, it's tofu that is the most familiar of the soyfood products.

Soy and Your Health

Somewhere along the way, people realized that the soybean—besides its protein content—had other nutritional benefits as well: it contains few saturated fats; has no cholesterol; and provides isoflavones, minerals, and fiber. Some believe that all these characteristics make soy an effective disease fighter, working hard to combat certain cancers, strokes, and heart disease. Some point out that, as a rule, Asians suffer from fewer of these diseases than Westerners, with their rich meaty diets, and they believe that soy consumption is one reason for that. Other studies suggest that soy's properties may also combat osteoporosis, type 2 diabetes, and even obesity.

But, as it turns out, while some people describe soy as a "miracle" food, some skeptics challenge the prevalent notion that soy should be a staple in everyone's diet, replacing meat partially or totally. If you scroll through the web, you'll find plenty of conflicting arguments about the pros and cons of soy that will leave you completely mystified.

Soy Is Good for You

In a 1999 ruling, the FDA allowed food manufacturers to label their soy-based food—foods made with the whole soybean without any added fats and that contain at least 6.25 grams of soy protein per serving—as beneficial for keeping hearts healthy. That approval apparently opened the floodgates of soy's popularity, and production of soyfoods soared.

In a 2000 *FDA Consumer* magazine article entitled "Soy: Health Claims for Soy Protein, Questions about Other Components," author John Henkel pinpoints the various health benefits of soy in the diet, stating that soy is a good substitute for animal protein because it is a complete protein, containing all the amino acids humans require without high levels of saturated fats. Referring to earlier studies, the author also notes that research suggests that soy proteins may lower the bad cholesterol levels in blood without affecting good cholesterol levels. In addition, eating soy may reduce the incidence of osteoporosis and certain cancers—studies were underway to determine soy's efficacy in these conditions.

Following the FDA's endorsement of soy and its possible benefits, the American Heart Association issued an advisory recommending soy products, with their polyunsaturated fats and fiber and low saturated fat, as possibly beneficial as a source of protein.

Soy Is Not Good for You

On the other side of the soy debate, soy detractors point out that eating soy not only has drawbacks, but also could have serious health effects. Some consumers have claimed that soy in infant formulas lowers IQ; others say soy causes thyroid problems.

The FDA itself in its 2000 article on soy confirmed that the jury may still be out for much of soy's touted health claims, particularly relating to soy isoflavones, which are a weak form of estrogen and in high levels could increase the risk of breast cancer; however, a study published by the *Cancer Project News* in 2006 and conducted by the Johns Hopkins School of Medicine found that high soy intake actually reduced breast cancer risk, particularly for premenopausal women.

An additional soy detractor is the D.C.-based Weston A. Price Foundation, which has filed a petition with the FDA asking the government agency to amend its earlier pro-soy statements. The petition suggests that soy may play a role in promoting certain cancers, in initiating thyroid diseases, and causing reproductive problems. It cites that the to-date scientific findings about soy's health benefits are inconclusive. For more information, visit *www.westonaprice.org*.

Additionally, the American Heart Association's Nutrition Committee, after reviewing twenty-two studies, is slightly revising its earlier statement about soy intake and its relationship to heart disease. Its conclusion: soy protein reduced harmful cholesterol by only 3 percent and had virtually no effect on lowering blood pressure. The committee's report added that the findings on soy protein's worth in preventing or treating breast or prostate cancers is not established. But researchers did note that using various soy products with their polyunsaturated fats to replace high-fat proteins had dietary benefit.

Many people report allergic reactions to soy proteins, a fact substantiated by the Asthma and Allergy Foundation of America, which reports that soy is one of the most common allergens in the market. It also notes that not all soyfoods cause a reaction, but since soy is now prevalent in many food products, even if the label does not state that soy is present, avoiding soy for the allergy sufferer becomes a challenge.

Draw Your Own Conclusions

As in all cases, the informed consumer is the best consumer. It's reasonable to assume that many of the modern soy products are not produced, formulated, or processed in the way the ancient Chinese and Japanese soy masters made their tofu. Therefore, you should select soyfoods that are basically whole soy or based on soy proteins, without overprocessing or many added ingredients: as a consumer, figure out the many ways to bring soy to your table. And as with all foods—and with anything in life—moderation is the key.

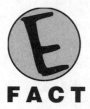

FACT

Controversial in today's marketplace are the development and marketing of GMO versus non-GMO foods. Simply stated, GMO crops have been genetically modified to achieve a particular goal, such as resistance to disease or pests. But opponents believe that science still does not have clear data about if or how such modification might in the long run upset the balance of nature and affect both the plant and animal kingdoms. Soybeans are one of the plants usually modified.

All about Tofu

Tofu is a white, bland-to-tasteless, odorless food that in its block form resembles cheese; when it is fermented, tofu may go by the nickname of "Chinese cheese," or less becomingly, "stinky tofu." But plain white tofu is perhaps the most recognized and cooked-with form of the processed soybean.

From Soybean to Tofu

So how did the soybean become tofu, or bean curd, or *doufou*, tofu's other names? One piece of folklore points back to a Han dynasty (later Han Dynasty, A.D. 25–220) cook who stumbled upon this food quite by accident when he mixed unrefined sea salt, which contains a natural coagulant, with a porridge of cooked soybeans and found the mixture coagulated. Chinese food historian E. N. Anderson shuns that tale, pointing to the late Tang or early Sung dynasties (A.D. 907–1209) as the most likely time frame.

Still other versions persist, but no matter which tale is true, the important point is that bean curd, or tofu, was born. And when they discovered it, vegetarian Buddhists quickly embraced this soybean product as a fine meat substitute—and tofu eventually found its way from China to Japan and then to much of the rest of the world.

In its earliest Chinese days, *doufou* was a peasant food, much desired as a source of low-cost protein. But it seems that a Ching dynasty emperor (the dynasty began in A.D. 1644) discovered *doufou* when wandering in one of the provinces, and thenceforth, bean curd became court food.

As if by magic, the white blocks of tofu have been transformed into various tofu products: the silken tofus, reflecting the Japanese way of processing the soybeans; the dried tofu sheets known as bean curd "skins" popular in Buddhist Chinese vegetarian cooking; fermented tofu; fried tofu; puffed tofu; dried tofu; flavored tofu; and tofus available in very soft, soft, firm, and extra-firm textures. That's a plus for modern cooks, who like to experiment in the kitchen with assorted tofu products.

If you have the desire, patience, and skills, you can even make tofu at home. The soybeans require lengthy soaking, then grinding and further processing. Or you can use soymilk plus a coagulant and strain the mixture for a speedier process. A faster way to make tofu, though, is to order a tofu-making kit or machine and follow directions. And the fastest way of all: use the Japanese-made instant tofu mix made from soymilk powder and other ingredients: just add water and stir.

Other Soyfood Products

If tofu is not at the top of your soy list, settle back and enjoy numerous other soy-based foods that should round out your menu. Most are readily available —many are already processed and cooked into ready-to-use products such as chili or hamburgers—and certainly easy to cook with. Soy products include the following:

- **Soy sauce:** Made from fermented soybeans, soy sauce is available as the traditional Chinese or Japanese soy sauce and also as tamari, a rich-flavored Japanese soy sauce made without wheat. Because of its sodium content, soy sauce is now available in low-sodium types—but some purists might not find the flavor as fully developed. The Malaysians and Indonesians also use thick, dark sweet or salty soy sauces in their cooking.

- **Tempeh:** An Indonesian soybean-and-grain product, tempeh is made by injecting the mixture with a mold, and after fermenting, the product has a salty flavor. It needs steaming, simmering, or frying before eating.

- **Miso:** A thick fermented and salted soybean paste ranging in color from white to dark brown, miso has been a Japanese staple from ancient times. It comes in hundreds of varieties, letting cooks select how they want to season stews, soups, dressings, and other foods. Miso requires lengthy aging and because it curdles if overheated, should be added to the cookpot at the end of cooking.

- **Edamame:** Shelled or still in the pod, edamame—fresh soybeans—can be readily found fresh and ready to eat or frozen at most well-stocked supermarkets. Although these are considered a Japanese food, the Chinese also enjoy edamame and call them *maodou*. According to the Soyfoods Council, the green soybean we know as edamame is actually just one of several soybean varieties. Edamame have long been enjoyed by the Japanese as a snack food.

- **Soybean sprouts:** Often mistaken for the smaller and tenderer mung bean sprouts, soybean sprouts are available at Asian markets, but rarely at Western ones. These are good in stir-fries.

- **Soy "meat" alternatives:** Meat alternatives from soy proteins combined with other ingredients, these products are meatlike—some even resemble seafood—in their appearance but not in their fat content. Many markets and health food groceries stock an array of these alternatives, such as soy "meat" crumbles, "sausages," deli slices, "hot dogs," "meatballs," and "bacon," as well as already-made meatlike dishes, such as chili. Although not really a meat analog, another soy product known as TVP, or texturized vegetable protein, is made from soy flour and cooks up quickly in dishes as a meat substitute.

- **Soymilk:** Made from soaked and ground soybeans, soymilks have proliferated, so you'll even find unsweetened and sweetened soymilk; chocolate, vanilla, and green tea soymilk; nonfat and low-fat soymilk; and soymilk in regular or aseptic packaging; the latter does not require refrigeration before using.
- **Soy dairy-free products:** It seems that each day a new soy dairy-free product hits the market. Vegetarians and vegans—and those who want a different kind of eating experience—enjoy soy cheeses in slices and shreds, yogurt (cultured soy), dairy-free frozen dessert, margarine, soy sour cream, and soy cream cheese. The cheeses come in many different flavors, from Cheddar to mozzarella.
- **Soy nuts:** Enjoyed like roasted cocktail nuts, soy nuts are either roasted or fried; some are seasoned and even coated in chocolate.
- **Soy mayonnaise:** This product resembles the standard mayonnaise, but without the eggs. You can make your own at home—look for recipes on the Internet.

Soy in the Kitchen

With all the soy-based products at hand, home cooks may want to know how to handle them. As the Soyfoods Association of North America (*www .soyfoods.org*) points out, you can work more soy into your diet and easily substitute the various soy ingredients for other ingredients, with some exceptions. One of these is soy flour, which contains no gluten, hence it cannot totally replace wheat flour in yeast-raised baked goods.

You can get a good handle of soy's culinary uses by referencing this website: *www.thesoyfoodscouncil.compdf/soy101/pdf.* And based on information by the Soyfoods Association of North America, you can pick up helpful tips about using these common soy-based foods:

- **Tofu:** As a perishable food, tofu needs refrigeration, unless you use the Japanese tofu packaged in aseptic vacuum-sealed cartons, which have a shelf life marked on the box. Otherwise, plan to use all other tofu within a few days, changing the water it's packed in daily to keep it fresh. You can also freeze fresh tofu, which gives it a chewier texture. Be sure you select the proper type of tofu for your intended recipe: all water-packed tofus—whether soft or extra-firm in texture, can stand up to stir-frying and other rigorous handling without falling apart; it also absorbs flavors well, making it a welcome addition to grilling and other dishes that profit from layers of flavors. The silken tofu, on the other hand, is a fragile substance that easily falls apart and is ideal for puréeing; it does not absorb flavors.

- **Tempeh:** Unless the package is marked "precooked," tempeh needs cooking—and most methods work well with tempeh—before use.
- **Soymilk:** Soymilk is available in the refrigerator case and on shelves in aseptic cartons. Once the carton is opened, the soymilk is perishable, so it needs refrigeration. Use unsweetened and unflavored soymilk for soups and savory dishes; sweetened and flavored soymilk is fine for desserts and smoothies. You can substitute soymilk in a one-to-one ratio for dairy milk. Be sure to shake the container before using the soymilk.
- **Soy dairy products:** All are perishable products, so require refrigeration. Note that soy cheeses handle differently than dairy cheeses, and in general, do not have the same melting characteristics. Soy sour cream is great for dips, but doesn't work well when heated; soy cream cheese and soy yogurt may be used as their dairy counterparts.
- **Soy "meat" alternatives:** Treat them as perishable foods and refrigerate or freeze them, as specified on the package.

400 calories
17g fat
30g carbohydrates
37g protein
460mg sodium
12g fiber

INGREDIENTS:

3 tablespoons vegetable oil

1 large onion, diced

1½ tablespoons minced garlic, or to taste

1½ tablespoons minced fresh ginger

1 tablespoon black bean–garlic paste

6 ounces soy "meat" crumbles

1 (10-ounce) package fresh edamame, rinsed

1 cup crumbled silken firm tofu

1 cup vegetable broth, or more as desired

1 tablespoon soy sauce, or more to taste

1 teaspoon toasted sesame oil, or more to taste

1 teaspoon crushed red pepper, or more as desired

Toasted soybeans for garnish

Sliced scallions for garnish

Diced firm tofu for garnish

Asian Soy Chili

For a totally Asian meal, consider serving this chili over hot steamed jasmine rice.

1. Heat the oil in a large saucepan over medium heat and sauté the onion, garlic, and ginger for 2 to 3 minutes or until fragrant. Stir in the black bean–garlic paste and the soy "meat" crumbles. Sauté for about 4 minutes.

2. Reduce the heat to medium-low. Stir in the edamame, tofu, broth, soy sauce, sesame oil, and crushed red pepper. Cook and stir for about 10 minutes. Serve in individual bowls, garnishing as desired.

Creamy Fruit Pudding

This simple pudding whips together quickly and has a cloudlike texture. If you eat it immediately, it will be soft, but it will firm up slightly after chilling for several hours. If you would prefer, use vanilla wafers instead of graham crackers for the cookie crust.

1. Combine the tofu, sour cream, soymilk, and pudding in a food processor or blender and purée. Add the vanilla extract, salt, and berries and purée again until smooth. You may need to do this in two batches.

2. Spread the graham cracker crumbs in a 2-quart dessert bowl and spoon the pudding mixture over top. Chill.

SERVES 4

440 calories
15g fat
62g carbohydrates
16g protein
590mg sodium
4g fiber

INGREDIENTS:

1 pound lite silken tofu, well-drained
1 (12-ounce) container soy sour cream
¾ cup soymilk or nonfat milk
1 (1½-ounce) box instant vanilla pudding
1 tablespoon vanilla extract
Pinch salt
2 cups frozen mixed berries
2 cups crushed graham crackers

SERVES 2

410 calories
32g fat
7g carbohydrates
22g protein
800mg sodium
2g fiber

INGREDIENTS:

2 tablespoons olive oil
1 teaspoon minced garlic
1 bunch scallions, trimmed and cut into 1-inch pieces
½ cup shelled edamame
1 tablespoon soy sauce, or to taste
3 large eggs
½ cup shredded regular or soy Cheddar cheese
Snips of fresh cilantro for garnish

Edamame Omelet

The addition of cheese turns this into a fusion dish; to add more Asian flavors, you might want to stir in some shredded daikon and crushed chiles to taste into the mix.

1. Heat 2 tablespoons oil in a small skillet over medium heat and sauté the garlic and scallion for about 2 minutes. Add the edamame and soy sauce and sauté 1 minute more. Remove from the skillet and set aside.

2. Heat the remaining 1 tablespoon oil in the same skillet. Beat the eggs until mixed and pour into the hot oil. Scatter the shredded cheese on top. Lift up the edges of the omelet, tipping the skillet back and forth to cook the uncooked eggs. When the top looks firm, sprinkle the scallion mixture over one half of the omelet and fold the other half over top.

3. Carefully lift the omelet out of the skillet. Divide it in half, sprinkle with the cilantro, and serve.

Soy Caesar Salad

The classic recipe contains a coddled egg that is "cooked" by the action of the lemon juice. Substituting mayonnaise provides the same creamy effect. For the best results, use only fresh lemon juice.

1. Discard the large, tough outer leaves and tear the remaining lettuce leaves into bite-sized pieces; discard the tough spines. Toss the leaves with the tofu puffs, the soy nuts, and 2 tablespoons Parmesan cheese.

2. Combine the olive oil and garlic in a small bowl and whisk briskly with a fork until the olive oil and garlic become well mixed. Whisk in the vinegar, mayonnaise, lemon juice, Worcestershire sauce, dry mustard, salt, and pepper. When the dressing is well mixed, whisk in the remaining 2 tablespoons cheese. Dress the salad, tossing to combine.

What Are Tofu Puffs?

If you haven't discovered these light-as-air squares of deep-fried tofu, add them to your shopping list the next time you go to an Asian market. While they may be a bit oily—some people say to boil them first to remove the excess oil—they act like sponges and soak up all the flavors of the sauce, curries, stews, and soups they cook in, in this case, the salad dressing. With their squishy texture, they are really addictive.

**SERVES 4 AS A
SIDE SALAD**

440 calories
38g fat
15g carbohydrates
15g protein
190mg sodium
3g fiber

INGREDIENTS:

*1 head romaine lettuce, rinsed
    and chilled
2 ounces tofu puffs, diced
1 cup toasted soy nuts
¼ cup soy Parmesan cheese, or
    more to taste
8 tablespoons olive oil, or more
    as needed
4 cloves garlic, minced
2 tablespoons red wine vinegar
2 tablespoons soy mayonnaise
1 tablespoon fresh lemon juice
1 teaspoon vegetarian
    Worcestershire sauce, or
    more to taste
1 teaspoon dry mustard
Salt and freshly ground black
    pepper to taste*

Asian Cabbage Stew with Tofu Puffs

To underscore this stew's Asian character, you could garnish it with crushed chow mein noodles and a handful of the Japanese snack food, wasabi-coated peas.

1. Heat the oil in a large saucepan over medium heat and sauté the garlic. Add the napa cabbage and the bok choy and sauté for 2 to 3 minutes.

2. Add the vegetable broth, tofu puffs, soy sauce, and chili-garlic sauce. Reduce the heat to low and cook until the cabbage is softened.

SERVES 4

320 calories
17g fat
31g carbohydrates
15g protein
730mg sodium
12g fiber

INGREDIENTS:

3 tablespoons vegetable oil
4 to 5 cloves garlic, mashed
1 head napa cabbage, cored and coarsely chopped
2 heads baby bok choy, rinsed and leaves separated
1 quart vegetable or mushroom broth
1 (4-ounce) package tofu puffs
Soy sauce to taste
Vietnamese chili-garlic sauce to taste

Ma Po Tofu

This dish has numerous variations, and this one showcases tofu with a backdrop of plenty of garlic and ginger; you can adjust the chili heat to suit your taste, and always feel free to add more garlic. Look for the black bean garlic sauce condiment at an Asian grocery or a well-stocked supermarket. Serve this over steamed rice.

1. Heat a large wok or skillet over medium heat and add the vegetable oil. When it is hot, add the garlic and the ginger and stir-fry for 30 seconds. Stir in the black bean garlic sauce, the soy sauce, and the chili paste.

2. Mix the vegetable stock together with the cornstarch and sugar and stir into the wok. Stir in the tofu and the soy "meat" and stir-fry the mixture until the sauce thickens and the tofu is heated through. Add the scallions, stir-fry for 1 to 2 minutes more, and serve.

SERVES 4

430 calories
22g fat
26g carbohydrates
44g protein
720mg sodium
10g fiber

INGREDIENTS:

3 tablespoons vegetable oil
4 cloves garlic, minced
1-inch piece fresh ginger, thinly sliced
3 tablespoons black bean–garlic sauce
2 tablespoons soy sauce
1 tablespoon Vietnamese garlic-chili paste, or more to taste
1 cup vegetable stock
1 tablespoon cornstarch
1 tablespoon sugar
1 pound firm tofu, drained, pressed dry, and diced
6 ounces soy "meat" crumbles
2 bunches scallions, trimmed and cut on the diagonal

SERVES 1

460 calories
31g fat
33g carbohydrates
18g protein
980mg sodium
8g fiber

INGREDIENTS:

1 tablespoon vegetable oil
3 ounces soy chorizo or other soy "sausage," formed into a patty
1 tablespoon soy cream cheese, softened to room temperature
2 slices whole-grain bread, toasted
Soy cheese slices, as desired

Soy Sandwich

Soy cheese slices are available in several different flavors. Make a selection that will complement the type of "sausage" you use. If you do not use the chorizo "sausage", you may want to sprinkle the patty with your favorite seasoning salt.

1. Heat the oil in a small skillet over medium heat and pan-fry the "sausage" patty until it is browned on both sides.

2. Spread the cream cheese on both slices of toast and lay on the "cheese" slices on the bottom slice. Top with the patty, close the sandwich, and enjoy.

Spicy Fried Bean Curd with Peanut Sauce

This flavorful dish takes the favorite Thai peanut sauce—traditionally used as a satay dipping sauce—and turns it into the basis for a spunky tofu dish. But in this variation, tofu becomes a star player in the dish.

1. To make the Peanut Sauce, pour the oil into a large skillet and heat over medium heat. Add the two curry pastes, the peanuts, and the coconut milk. Heat till mixture comes to a boil, then add sugar and tamarind juice, reduce the heat to low, and cook, stirring often, until the mixture thickens into a sauce.

2. Meanwhile, slice the pressed tofu into 6 uniform blocks and dust them thoroughly on all sides in cornstarch. Heat the oil in a large wok and when the oil is hot, add the tofu pieces, one at a time. Cook the tofu on the first side until the bottoms have turned golden and puffy. Gently turn the pieces over, adding more oil if needed, and fry the second sides until golden. Remove from the wok and drain on paper towels.

3. Spoon the Peanut Sauce into a large bowl and arrange the tofu on a serving platter. Pass the sauce and tofu.

What Are Palm Sugar and Tamarind Juice?

Palm sugar is a creamy-colored brown sugar that is the sap from one of two different palms. It produces a gentler sweetness than the Western brown sugar, which is an option if you cannot find palm sugar. Tamarind juice is the liquid that forms after soaking the pulp from the tamarind pod and squeezing out the liquid. It adds a sweet-sour taste to Thai dishes. People will try to tell you that lime or lemon juices are substitutes; they definitely are not. Fortunately, tamarind pulp and juice are easy to find in Asian markets.

SERVES 4 TO 6

600 calories
39g fat
52g carbohydrates
22g protein
55mg sodium
5g fiber

INGREDIENTS:

Peanut Sauce:

1 tablespoon vegetable oil
3 tablespoons Thai red curry paste
1 tablespoon Thai Mussaman curry paste
2 cups chopped fresh-roasted peanuts
1 cup coconut milk
1 cup palm sugar or brown sugar
1 cup tamarind juice

Fried Tofu

1 (1 pound) block extra-firm tofu, drained and pressed dry
Cornstarch for coating
¼ to ½ cup vegetable oil for frying

Mediterranean Tofu

SERVES 4

290 calories
18g fat
23g carbohydrates
12g protein
650mg sodium
5g fiber

INGREDIENTS:

2 tablespoons vegetable oil
1 large sweet onion, diced
4 cloves garlic, minced
3 zucchini, thinly sliced
*1 (14½-ounce) can crushed
    tomatoes*
*1 (1 pound) package silken firm
    tofu, cubed*
1 cup pitted kalamata olives

*Because you are using silken tofu, it will partially fall apart as
you stir the dish, dispersing itself throughout the mixture.*

1. Heat the oil in a large wok or skillet and sauté the onion and garlic for about 3 minutes.

2. Add the zucchini and cook 3 minutes more.

3. Add the tomatoes, tofu, and olives and cook 2 to 3 minutes more. Serve.

Miso Soup with Soba Noodles and Fried Tofu

Japan's beloved miso soup typically contains little bits of cubed tofu. But in this variation, tofu becomes a star player in the dish.

1. Bring a pot of lightly salted water to a boil and cook the soba noodles; these cook quickly, so test them for doneness after about 3 minutes. Drain and toss them to separate the strands.

2. Bring 6 cups water to a boil and stir in the miso paste; start gradually so you find the right flavor for you. When it is fully dissolved, add the tofu and continue cooking until the tofu is heated. Add the watercress leaves.

3. Portion the noodles into 4 soup bowls and ladle the hot soup over the noodles. Add soy sauce, as desired, and serve.

SERVES 4

290 calories
13g fat
32g carbohydrates
16g protein
590mg sodium
3g fiber

INGREDIENTS:

4 ounces dry soba noodles
3 tablespoons miso paste, or to taste
1 (9-ounce) package fried tofu, diced
1 bunch watercress, leaves only
Soy sauce to taste

CHAPTER 11

The World of Pastas

"Life is a combination of magic and pasta," a quote attributed to Federico Fellini, speaks volumes about the mystical bond between water, flour, salt, and sometimes egg. This bond results in a dough that, when cooked, glorifies even the humblest table. You can say all you want about carbs, no carbs, strict diets, and epicurean meals, but when the dust clears, you find the finest comfort food in the world is probably pasta.

Perfectly Pasta

When you stop to think about it, what other staple has universal appeal equal to pasta's? This shaped—and sometimes colored and enriched—dough turns up in some form in almost every country. Traditionally, it appears in Germany's and Tibet's dumplings, Spain's noodle-based paella, North Africa's couscous, and India's vermicelli-based dessert, for example. Where pasta is not native to the cuisine, pasta fanciers are beginning to demand this versatile staple, making pasta a global favorite.

If economy counts as one factor for pasta's popularity, its versatility matters as well. According to the Washington, D.C.-based National Pasta Association, pasta comes in hundreds of shapes and numerous colors including red (beets tomatoes), green (spinach), and black (squid ink), and pasta is so versatile that cooks can boil, steam, fry, or bake it. Pasta's mild flavor partners well with numerous fillings and toppings and with every sort of beverage, from champagne and red wine to hot tea and chilled lemonade. Americans love pasta so much they eat about 4.3 pounds per person per year.

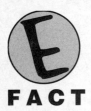

FACT

A 1997 survey conducted for the National Pasta Association, concluded that residents of the Northeast were more likely than people in other parts of the country to eat pasta on a weekly basis, while Southerners were less likely to eat pasta regularly. However, the most dramatic increase in pasta consumption overall was in the South, where 42 percent of Southerners are eating more pasta today than they were five years ago.

Savvy consumers appreciate its good value per serving and also applaud its nutritional benefits. Pasta fanciers can find not only whole-grain pastas, but also varieties that are gluten free, made from artichokes and quinoa, or enriched with eggs and with omega-3 fatty acids. And, the USDA, with its FoodPyramid, cites pasta as a valuable nutrient-dense food, urging Americans to include at least three ounces of whole-grain pasta (or other grains) each day.

A Pasta Primer

If you are like most consumers, instead of getting down to basics you probably just pick up a box of Italian-style dried pasta, select a prepared sauce, and head home with your purchases for a simple pasta meal. But to maximize your pasta pleasure, learn a few basic facts.

Italian Pastas

Thanks to the ingenuity of countless Italian cooks and chefs over the centuries, pasta now appears in hundreds of different shapes. In general, you can use most shapes interchangeably, but a rule of thumb is this: shaped pastas work best with chunky sauces; long, thin strands with smooth sauces; and flat shapes with layering.

While many pasta shapes remain regional in parts of Italy, consumers can count on readily finding many pasta basics at their supermarkets, including the following:

- **Spaghetti:** The long, thin tubular pasta known as spaghetti is perhaps the most familiar one to American consumers. It is available in several thicknesses, and thus may be called spaghetti, vermicelli, spaghettini, bucatini, or fedellini, depending on its thickness.
- **Elbow macaroni:** Who doesn't know the short tubular pasta known as macaroni? It lends itself well to many different recipes and cooking techniques.
- **Lasagna:** These broad, flat pasta sheets are traditionally used as layering for many kinds of fillings; some markets now stock a version of "fast" lasagna sheets that don't need precooking before the layering process. Lasagna-based dishes are economical and may be as simple or fancy as the cook chooses.
- **Fusilli:** Long, slender twists that if straight, would be spaghetti. Fusilli may be used as is or broken into shorter pieces for salads and soups.
- **Shells:** Available in varying sizes, shells capture and hold chunky sauces, and the largest shells are perfect for filling with cheeses and vegetables and topping with a sauce for a baked entrée. These are made with whole wheat or refined flours.

- **Orzo:** Shaped like grains of rice—or as other see it, like barley pearls—this small pasta adds texture to soups but also works well in salads and baked dishes.
- **Ravioli**: Round or square pasta pillows encasing a savory—and sometimes, sweet—filling. Fresh ravioli are readily available in most supermarkets and make a satisfying first or main course meal with a variety of different toppings.

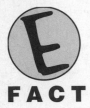

FACT

Novelty pasta shapes also take their place on the market shelf. Some of these are traditional; others are not. These include the kid-favorite alphabet pastas; the rotelli, shaped like wheels; and those made for special occasions or special interest groups, such as the pasta shaped like Christmas trees or pumpkins.

Asian Pastas

Thanks to the proliferation of Asian cooking, Asian ingredients, and Asian restaurants across the nation, many consumers are now familiar with assorted Asian pastas, probably the most familiar being the medium-thin rice noodles used for cooking pad Thai. Also common are Chinese dumplings; Japanese noodle soups based on thick udon noodles; the Japanese ramen noodles, now available dried and vacuum-packed for instant meals; and the Southeast Asian bean thread, or cellophane, noodles made popular as a Hollywood fad-diet staple. All have brought the world of Asian noodles into the marketplace.

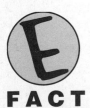

FACT

Ramen noodles are so popular they merit their own museum in Yokohama, Japan, and their own website, *www.ramenlicious.com*.

Unlike their Western counterparts, Asian pastas may be made from wheat, rice, buckwheat, seaweed, tapioca starch, devil's tongue yam starch, and mung bean starch, and they may be flavored with green tea or spinach. If you have an Asian market nearby, check out the numerous fresh and dried varieties for sale on shelves as fully stocked as any pasta section in a Western market. The most prevalent Asian pastas include:

- **Rice noodles:** Made from rice flour and water and extruded in various thicknesses, from the very thin rice vermicelli to the thick Vietnamese and Thai rice ribbons, these are as easy to cook with as Western pastas. These noodles work well in many kinds of recipes, from soups and salads to curry entrées. If you are lucky, you may find an Asian market that stocks the fresh wide rice ribbon noodles, delicious when quick-rinsed in hot water and topped with a savory mixture.

- **Asian or Chinese wheat noodles:** Sold dry or, more often in Asian markets, fresh, these come in varying widths and cook up as easily as Western spaghetti. And like Western spaghetti, you should cook these in plenty of water; these require rinsing after cooking to prevent sticking together. Some varieties contain eggs, and the packages will note that. If you can't find these wheat noodles you can substitute spaghetti in your recipe. You'll also find the very slender egg noodles for stir-frying or making into a fried noodle "nest."

- **Somen noodles:** Thin, delicate wheat noodles favored in Japan for simple soups, these are often served chilled in hot weather and cook up quickly.

- **Soba noodles:** These darker buckwheat noodles have a rich almost nutty flavor and make a delicious basis for soups and salads.

- **Udon noodles:** White, slippery soba noodles, these vary in thickness, are often sold fresh in Asian markets, and are delicious in soups and stews.

- **Wonton or egg roll skins:** Simply sheets of rolled-out-flat pasta dough, these skins are very popular in China and elsewhere in Asia for wrapping up assorted fillings and then either steaming, boiling, or frying the end result. The skins are readily available fresh in most well-stocked supermarkets and may be either round or square.

Fresh Versus Dried

Probably every cook who makes pasta a part of his menu planning can weigh in on this topic, with differing opinions. Even the esteemed food magazine *Cook's Illustrated* dedicated an entire article to this controversy, concluding that whether you use dried or fresh pasta really depends on the kind of sauce you plan to use.

Delicate fresh pasta should be porous enough to absorb both sauce and flavor; dried pasta is firmer and better with thicker sauces. And finally, the article suggests that the fresh pastas you find at market have probably been idling in the refrigerator section for so long they are really no longer "fresh," and have likely lost the very freshness and texture quality people seek. Besides, the article notes, commercial fresh pastas don't have the same formula as homemade or chef-made fresh pastas.

Using a pasta-making machine or developing the skills for rolling out the dough means you can have your own fresh pasta—noodles, wrappers, certain shapes—whenever you get the time to make your own. The pasta dough is simple enough to mix with a food processor, and you'll find plenty of recipes for making egg, eggless, buckwheat, and whole wheat pastas. But selecting the right combination of ingredients for fresh dough is open to dispute: Whole eggs? Egg yolks? No eggs? Olive oil? Water? Wheat flour, whole wheat flour, or semolina? The choices seem almost infinite—and that's where the disagreements begin.

But when deciding between fresh and dried pasta, you should take other factors into consideration: fresh pastas cost more, and these need to be used up within a few days. Dried pastas, however, have an endless shelf life, unless wrapped and stored carelessly. And because their basic formula is different, dried pastas have a firmer texture that stands up to vigorous handling and a wider assortment of toppings and sauces.

Health Benefits of Pasta

As a staple with its own inherent health-promoting capacities, pasta has value as the carrier of nutritious and flavorful sauces and toppings. Putting that all together makes pasta a uniquely qualified component of vegetarian and nonvegetarian meals.

Pasta, the "Good" Carbohydrate

According to a 2007 report released by the International Pasta Organisation [sic], pasta is something of a wonder food when it is made from whole grains and thus a source of B vitamins and iron. Containing no cholesterol and being low in sodium, it makes a healthful component in everyone's diet, even those who need to control their dietary sugars. Pasta, in moderation, of course, can easily fit into a dieter's regimen: 1 cup of cooked pasta contains 200 calories; this figure varies depending on the pasta variety eaten.

And the National Pasta Association elaborates on pasta's nutritional benefits. Describing pasta as a complex carb, it points out that pasta is fortified with folic acid, an important B vitamin that not only helps the central nervous system, it also helps protect unborn babies against neurological problems. And it may help prevent heart disease in women.

Preparing Perfect Pasta

Faced with portions of either fresh or dried pasta, you must decide: what to do next? You should learn a few basic tips to be sure you always get it right. Few culinary missteps are as distressing as serving a plate of gummy, overcooked—or undercooked and tough—pasta.

Into the Pot

All kitchen experts agree: to achieve that perfect texture, you must cook pasta in at least four quarts of rapidly boiling, salted water—about one tablespoon of salt. The ratio of water to pasta should be about four to one. And the water must be boiling furiously or the pasta may stick together in the pot. After adding the pasta, most experts advise to briefly cover the pot to return the water to its rapid boil, removing the lid totally or partially once the water boils again.

But then the experts begin to disagree: to prevent sticking, to stir or not to stir; to add a little olive oil or not in the cooking water? Olive oil may prevent the pasta from sticking together, but as one source notes, it also may prevent the sauce from clinging in the finished dish.

The cooking times, too, vary from pasta to pasta; your best bet is to follow manufacturer's directions in timing. Obviously, fresh pastas cook faster. But the cooking time for dried pastas depends on its shape. After a few moments of cooking, you should test a piece of pasta to see if it has reached the desired al dente texture, that toothsome quality between tough and overcooked. If it hasn't, keep cooking and testing, and definitely avoid overcooking, or the pasta will likely lose its inherent texture.

When ready, drain the pasta in a colander, shaking it to remove extra water. Some authoritative sources say you should *never* rinse pasta in cold water. Rinsing, it seems, removes the starch part that helps sauces to stick to the pasta. Another opinion is that you may rinse pasta in cold water if you plan to use the pasta in a salad. Others recommend saucing the pasta right away, or at the very least, drizzling it lightly with olive oil to prevent sticking.

Garlicky Pasta Tossed with Sun-Dried Tomatoes

Select the most intriguing pasta shape and use it as a basis for this dish. Already roasted garlic cloves are sold at some markets.

1. Bring a large pot of lightly salted water to a boil and cook the pasta until al dente, 6 to 8 minutes. Drain and put into a large bowl.

2. Squeeze the cloves out of the roasted garlic and add to the bowl. Toss with the remaining ingredients and adjust seasonings.

Roasting Garlic

You'll find many suggestions for roasting garlic, but the simplest one is this: preheat the oven to 400°F, slice off about ¼ inch from the top, remove the outer papery skin, set the head or heads in a small heat-proof bowl, and drizzle the garlic with olive oil. Wrap the bowl in aluminum foil and roast for about 1 hour.

SERVES 2

750 calories
39g fat
71g carbohydrates
33g protein
690mg sodium
4g fiber

INGREDIENTS:

4 ounces dried shaped pasta
¼ cup oil-packed sun-dried
    tomatoes, slivered
1 whole head garlic, roasted and
    cooled
1 cup shredded fontina cheese
⅓ cup grated Parmesan cheese
3 tablespoons toasted pine nuts
1 tablespoon olive oil
Salt and freshly ground black
    pepper to taste

SERVES 4

750 calories
40g fat
85g carbohydrates
15g protein
970mg sodium
9g fiber

INGREDIENTS:

1 (17.6-ounce) package fresh
    gnocchi
1 bunch broccolini, chopped
    and cooked
10 baby purple potatoes, cooked
    and cubed
1 (13¾-ounce) can artichoke
    hearts, drained and
    quartered
3 tablespoons capers
½ cup olive oil
3 tablespoons red wine vinegar
2 tablespoons pesto
Salt and freshly ground black
    pepper to taste

Gnocchi and Purple Potatoes with Broccolini

*By garnishing this dish with a dusting of grated Parmesan
cheese or a portion of shredded mozzarella or fontina cheese,
you can achieve a different flavor profile. And for a kick of
heat, add sparingly some crushed red pepper.*

1. Cook the gnocchi according to package directions, drain, and put into a serving bowl. Add the broccolini, potatoes, artichoke hearts, and capers.

2. Whisk together the oil, vinegar, pesto, salt, and pepper. Pour over the vegetables and toss to combine. Serve.

What Are Gnocchi?

A knot-shaped pasta most commonly made with mashed potatoes and flour, gnocchi, when freshly made and right from the boiling water, are so delicate they seem to whisper. Another less common version is made with semolina flour, milk, and cheese. You can make potato gnocchi yourself, but fresh ones are sold at Italian markets and some supermarkets.

Cellophane Noodle Salad

SERVES 4

170 calories
1.5g fat
32g carbohydrates
9g protein
590mg sodium
3g fiber

In the traditional Thai version of this salad, cooks use fish sauce instead of soy sauce and use ground pork, shrimp, and/ or chicken for the meat. Thais also are likely to use dried "rat dropping" chiles that they crumble into the bowl. Mighty hot.

1. Drain the soaked and softened noodles and cut them into serving pieces. Put the noodles, "chicken" strips if using, scallions, cilantro leaves, and crushed red peppers into a serving bowl.
2. Mix together the lime juice, soy sauce, and pickled garlic and toss with the salad ingredients.

What Are Cellophane Noodles?

Called "glass," "cellophane," or "bean thread" noodles, this Asian pasta is made from the starch of mung beans, and when dried, the noodles are so brittle and tough that when you cut them—and the cleanest way is using scissors—they may fly around, so hold them over the sink. They are easier to cut when wet, although when they are wet they are also somewhat gelatinous. Unless you plan to use the softened noodles in a soup, drain them before using them in other dishes. These are readily available at most well-stocked supermarkets and at Asian markets.

INGREDIENTS:

4 ounces cellophane, or bean thread, noodles, softened in hot water for 20 minutes

1 (6-ounce) package soy "chicken" strips, optional

½ cup thinly sliced scallions

½ cup fresh cilantro leaves

1 to 2 tablespoons crushed red peppers

2 tablespoons lime juice

2 tablespoons soy sauce

1 tablespoon pickled garlic, chopped

Sugar to taste

SERVES 4

170 calories
1g fat
37g carbohydrates
4g protein
20mg sodium
3g fiber

INGREDIENTS:

*3 cups mixed young salad
  greens
2 cups cooked small shells.
  cooled
1 cup thinly sliced fresh
  strawberries
1 cup halved grapes
3 tablespoons plain yogurt
2 tablespoons balsamic vinegar
2 tablespoons honey, or to taste
Mint leaves for garnish*

Summer Salad with Shells

*Although shells make an attractive pasta base, feel free to
substitute another small pasta of your choice. You may also
use a fruit-flavored yogurt for additional flavor interest.*

1. Toss the greens with the shells, strawberries, and grapes and set
   aside.

2. Whisk together the yogurt, vinegar, and honey and toss with the
   salad ingredients. Before serving, garnish the salad with the mint
   leaves.

Mexi Mac 'n' Cheese

*This grown-up version of mac 'n' cheese rouses people with its
fiery bite. You can kick this up a notch or two by adding both
jalapeño and habanero chiles as a garnish. But you may need
a fire extinguisher.*

1. Preheat the oven to 350°F. Layer 2 cups taco chips on the bottom of
   a 2-quart heatproof dish.

2. Cook the macaroni in lightly salted water until al dente. Drain and
   set aside.

3. Meanwhile, melt the butter and whisk in the flour and milk, stirring
   for a few minutes until the mixture begins to thicken and is lump
   free. Stir in the salsa, Cheddar cheese, salt, and pepper. Combine
   the pasta with the cheese sauce and spoon into the prepared dish.
   Top with the remaining chips, the habanero cheese, and jalapeño
   slices.

4. Bake for about 30 minutes or until the cheese is melted throughout.
   Serve with softened flour tortillas.

SERVES 6

640 calories
32g fat
62g carbohydrates
25g protein
960mg sodium
3g fiber

INGREDIENTS:

3 cups crushed taco chips
8 ounces elbow macaroni
3 tablespoons butter
3 tablespoons flour
2 cups milk
1 cup hot or mild salsa
*2 cups shredded Cheddar
cheese*
*Salt and freshly ground black
pepper to taste*
*4 ounces habanero cheese,
cubed*
Jalapeño slices to taste
Flour tortillas for serving

600 calories
14g fat
111g carbohydrates
14g protein
40mg sodium
12g fiber

INGREDIENTS:
*1 (10-ounce) box quick-cooking
    couscous*
1 cup chopped flat-leaf parsley
1 cup cashews
½ cup raisins
½ cup cubed dried papaya
½ cup chopped dates
½ cup diced dried figs
½ cup chopped dried apricots
3 kiwifruit, peeled and sliced
½ red onion, diced
*1 (6-ounce) container nonfat
    lime yogurt*
2 tablespoons balsamic vinegar
1 tablespoon olive oil
Creole seasoning salt to taste
Mint leaves for garnish

Couscous Fruit and Nut Salad

*Don't be alarmed by the long list of ingredients. This salad
comes together in minutes, and it bursts with so much flavor
and texture, you will want to serve it often.*

1. Cook the couscous according to package directions and when it is cool add to the salad bowl.

2. Meanwhile, add the parsley, cashews, raisins, papaya, dates, figs, apricots, kiwifruit, and red onion to the bowl and stir to combine.

3. Whisk together the yogurt, vinegar, and olive oil and toss with the salad ingredients. Season with the Creole seasoning salt, garnish with mint leaves, and serve.

What Is Kiwifruit?
A fuzzy, small, oval fruit, the kiwifruit is a native of New Zealand and apparently was named after the country's national pride, the kiwi bird. Its inner green flesh contains little black seeds and offers a bright, slightly tart flavor. It's also commonly just called "kiwi" outside of New Zealand.

Cannellini and Tortellini

For a splash of color, add some chopped-up oil-packed sundried tomatoes to taste. Additionally, you can boost flavors with a garnish of capers and pitted niçoise olives.

1. Cook the tortellini according to package directions, drain, and set aside.

2. Meanwhile, heat the oil in a large skillet over medium heat and sauté the garlic and the "meatballs" for 4 to 5 minutes. Add the cannellini and tomatoes and continue cooking until the mixture in heated through. Season with salt and pepper. Add the tortellini, stirring to combine, and serve.

SERVES 4

590 calories
20g fat
69g carbohydrates
33g protein
960mg sodium
9g fiber

INGREDIENTS:

1 (12-ounce) package fresh tortellini

3 tablespoons olive oil

5 cloves garlic, minced

1 (9-ounce) package soy "meatballs"

1 (19-ounce) can cannellini, drained and rinsed

1 (14½-ounce) can roasted tomatoes

Salt and freshly ground black pepper to taste

SERVES 4

340 calories
9g fat
50g carbohydrates
13g protein
1,210mg sodium
6g fiber

INGREDIENTS:

1½ ounces rice vermicelli, cooked and cooled

8 pieces red leaf lettuce, rinsed, dried, and trimmed to fit

½ cup julienned red bell pepper

12 sprigs fresh cilantro, rinsed

16 or more mint leaves, rinsed

1 (6-ounce) package soy "beef" strips

8 (6-inch round) rice paper wrappers

4 scallions, trimmed and sliced in half lengthwise

¾ cup hoisin sauce

3 tablespoons minced garlic

2 tablespoons lime juice

2 tablespoons crunchy peanut butter

1 tablespoon Vietnamese chili garlic sauce, or more to taste

Summer Rolls

The inspiration for the summer rolls comes from Vietnam, but this Americanized version calls for scallions instead of garlic chives and soy "beef" strips instead of shrimp or pork; the "beef" strips are ready to use without any cooking.

1. Divide the noodles, lettuce, red pepper, cilantro, mint leaves, and "beef" strips into 8 separate and uniform piles and set aside.

2. Sprinkle 2 sheets of rice paper at a time with water and when each softens and is pliable, place one piece of lettuce on the wrapper. Starting at the upper edge of the wrapper, layer on red pepper, cilantro, mint leaves, "beef" strips, and noodles about ½ inch down from the upper edge. Fold the top edge over the filling, and then fold the right side over the filling. Roll the rice paper toward you tightly, keeping the right edge folded in, making a packet with one open side. Slide 1 or 2 scallion pieces into the opening and set the roll aside. Repeat with remaining ingredients.

3. Arrange the rolls on a serving plate and keep them covered with moist paper towels until ready to eat.

4. Mix together the hoisin sauce, garlic, lime juice, peanut butter, and Vietnamese sauce, stirring well to mix in the peanut butter. Place in a serving dish and pass with the summer rolls.

What Are Rice Paper Wrappers?

Pastalike in their flexibility and much like Chinese eggroll or springroll wrappers, these paper-thin wrappers are made from a paste of rice flour and water—and sometimes a starch for added strength—and after rolling out, are traditionally dried on bamboo mats, hence the cross-hatch pattern. When using, be careful not to saturate the wrappers. Some recipes call for leaving them in the water for up to 1 minute to soak, others say to boil them; that will only ruin the wrappers. These soften quickly with just a quick rush under cold water or a sprinkling with cold water.

Thai Curry Noodles

The fresh egg noodles cook very quickly, within 1 minute or so; do not overcook. Cook the noodles when the curry mixture is almost ready so you can serve the noodles with the sauce right away.

1. Heat the oil in a large wok over medium heat and stir-fry the garlic for about 30 seconds. Add the curry paste, stirring to dissolve, and add the coconut milk and the sugar. Cook for another 2 to 3 minutes or until the mixture is well combined. Reduce the heat to medium-low and add the red pepper, tofu, and "beef" strips.

2. Meanwhile, bring a large pot of lightly salted water to a boil and cook the noodles for about 1 minute. Drain.

3. Pour the noodles into a big serving bowl and top with the curry mixture. Garnish with the cilantro and peanuts and serve.

What Is Thai Red Curry Paste?

Traditionally, Thais make this paste with plenty of dried red chile peppers, lemongrass, galangal, palm sugar, garlic, and shrimp paste. However, some brands available in the marketplace contain no shrimp paste or fish sauce. Be sure you read the label first. Note that this can be very hot to timid palates, so taste as you go.

SERVES 4

740 calories
62g fat
37g carbohydrates
21g protein
135mg sodium
7g fiber

INGREDIENTS:

3 tablespoons vegetable oil
4 cloves garlic, minced
2 tablespoons Thai red curry paste, or more to taste
3 cups coconut milk
2 tablespoons brown sugar, or to taste
1 sweet red pepper, julienned
1 (9-ounce) package fried tofu, diced
3 ounces soy "beef" strips
½ pound fresh Chinese egg noodles
Fresh cilantro leaves for garnish
Peanuts for garnish

Udon Noodle Slaw

SERVES 4

220 calories
7g fat
33g carbohydrates
7g protein
1,670mg sodium
2g fiber

INGREDIENTS:

1 (1 pound) package fresh udon
    noodles
6 ounces broccoli slaw
3 tablespoons pickled ginger
⅓ cup soy sauce
2 tablespoon brown rice vinegar
1 tablespoon toasted sesame oil
1 tablespoon mayonnaise
1 tablespoon sugar
Sprinkles of rice seasoning for
    garnish

*Make this dish ahead and chill it for an easy and refreshing
supper or light lunch. This is one cooked pasta that you'll want
to drain and rinse off in cold water. Otherwise, you'll find
starch clings to the strands.*

1. Bring a large pot of water to a boil and cook the noodles for about 1 minute. Drain and rinse in cold water. Set aside to cool slightly.

2. Add the broccoli slaw and the ginger to a salad bowl. Mix together the soy sauce, vinegar, sesame oil, mayonnaise, and sugar, stirring to combine well. Add the noodles to the bowl and toss the mixture together until well combined. Add the dressing and toss again. Sprinkle with rice seasoning and serve.

CHAPTER 12

Great Grains

Perhaps one of man's oldest foods, grains of every variety have sustained the human race, becoming the cornerstone of many diets. Few would argue with their inherent benefits: cooks find that grains heat up into a wealth of delicious meals; nutritionists urge people to follow a whole-grains diet to improve their health. For everyone, whole grains are a win-win foodstuff.

What Are Grains?

As a food group, grains include oats, barley, wheat, rye, brown rice, amaranth, buckwheat, millet, quinoa, and sorghum. All these grains—some are "pseudograins"—are eaten whole or processed into the various cereals, pastas, tortillas, and breads you eat.

Because of their inherent fragility, plants and their remains vanish over time. But one research group in an Israeli dig found solid evidence—well-preserved plant remains—dating back tens of thousands of years, suggesting that early man ate a variety of wild cereals and grasses. This suggests that cultivating various grains were the earliest attempts at farming.

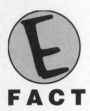

FACT

A pseudograin is a seed or kernel that is not a member of the grass family but is treated like a grain in the kitchen. According to the Wheat Foods Council, these include amaranth, flaxseed, quinoa, and buckwheat.

Refined Grains

As widely reported, grain products are divided into two categories: refined and whole grain. Food manufacturers refine whole grains by milling them and removing the bran, the endosperm, and the germ of the grain. Refining does yield a product with a finer texture and a longer shelf life, but during the milling process, many of the whole grains' nutrients and fiber are discarded.

After processing, manufacturers enrich the refined product by adding back some vitamins and iron, but the end result does not compare nutritionally to the original whole grains. You will find many refined-grains products in the marketplace, including flours, cereals, and pastas.

Whole Grains

Whole grains are just that: whole, with the bran, germ, and endosperm intact. Examples include brown rice, whole wheat flour, oats, and corn and whole cornmeal. For more information about whole grains, visit *www.whole grainscouncil.org*.

You don't have to hunt far to discover the benefits of keeping whole grains in your diet. As studies suggest, whole-grain foods are a rich source of B vitamins that provide energy to keep you active, plus other nutrients and fiber to enrich your health: they reduce the risk of heart disease, lower cholesterol, and protect against assorted diseases, including several chronic diseases. In addition, a recent study reported in the *American Journal of Clinical Nutrition* showed that men who ate a diet high in whole grains reduced their risk of developing type 2 diabetes.

Refined Versus Whole Grains

To understand the nutritional differences between whole wheat flour and refined and enriched white flours, study this chart from the USDA's 2005 Dietary Guidelines for Americans. Of course, whole wheat flours are not ideal for, or even suited to, baking fine pastries and cakes, but for everyday baked goods, using whole wheat or white whole wheat flour makes good nutritional sense:

COMPARISON OF 100 GRAMS OF WHOLE-GRAIN WHEAT FLOUR AND ENRICHED, BLEACHED, WHITE, ALL-PURPOSE FLOUR		
	100 Percent Whole-Grain Wheat Flour	**Enriched, Bleached, All-Purpose Flour**
Calories, kcal	339.0	364.0
Dietary Fiber, g	12.2	2.7
Calcium, mg	34.0	15.0
Magnesium, mg	138.0	22.0
Potassium, mg	405.0	107.0
Folate, DFE, mg	44.0	291.0
Thiamin, mg	0.05	.08
Riboflavin, mg	0.2	0.5
Niacin, mg	6.4	5.9
Iron, mg	3.9	4.6

Source: Agricultural Research Service Nutrient Database for Standard Reference, Release 17.

But using refined grains, particularly wheat, in the kitchen does have some practical implications: for one, white flour without the fatty germ doesn't tend to turn rancid, hence it lasts longer. Also white-flour products, especially breads and baked goods, have a finer texture; breads, in particular, tend to rise better without the germ and the bran.

What Grains Are You Eating?

Sadly, reports the USDA, while many Americans eat plenty of grains each day in the form of breads, tortillas, breakfast cereals, and pastas, few eat enough whole-grains foods. According to their standards, at least half of the grains—three ounces for a 2,000-calorie-a-day diet—eaten daily should be whole grains. That should include at least 28 grams of fiber daily, the amount recommended by the National Academy of Sciences/Institute of Medicine.

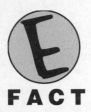

FACT

September is cited as whole-grains month, and to celebrate the occasion, the Whole Grains Council includes such events as a Whole Grains Challenge and a Whole Grains Giveaway. The focus of the council is to make Americans more aware of the health benefits of including whole grains in their diet.

If you are unsure of the whole-grain status of the foods you are buying, read the label. According to the FDA's labeling guidelines, for a product to be considered "whole-grain" it must contain at least 51 percent of whole-grain ingredients—in other words, "whole grain" comes first on the list. Similarly, a "100-percent whole-grain" product is labeled falsely if it contains other ingredients besides whole grains.

Adding Whole Grains to Your Diet

Embracing a whole-grains diet means keeping an eye on what goes in the grocery cart, and you can make simple changes without much effort. The first step: Whenever possible, pick up whole-grain products, including cereals, brown rice, and whole wheat pastas. Select whole-grain breads; make your own whole-grain or whole wheat baked goods; use whole grains as the basis for pilafs and stir-fries; and snack on whole-grain cookies, chips, or even popcorn, preferably unbuttered. For more ideas on getting the grains you need, look to *www.wholegrainscouncil.org*.

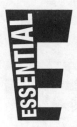

Want to know how many whole grains to fit in your diet? According to the USDA, that all depends on your age, sex, and activity level. To find out how much is enough, study the USDA chart at this site: *www.mypyramid .gov/pyramid/grains_amount.aspx#*.

Tips for Cooking Whole Grains

As with every other food group, whole grains in their natural state require some kitchen prep before getting to the cookpot. First, grains need rinsing in cold water to remove any dust or other particles; rinse until the water runs clear. Then, some sturdy whole grains such as farro, a wheat grain, benefit from soaking before cooking; the soaking of farro should last for about one hour, though some cooks tell you to soak farro overnight. Check your recipes for other soaking times.

In the cookpot, whole grains can steam, stir-fry with some liquid added, or boil then simmer to achieve their doneness. Many whole grains retain some chewiness when done. For cooking whole-grain products such as pasta, follow the package directions, being careful not to overcook the ingredient to the point of mushiness. Whole grains probably double in volume after cooking, thus yielding more than twice their original uncooked volume.

The Wheats

Food historians agree that wheat in its various forms may be one of mankind's oldest foods, but just where wheat growing and eating first originated is disputed. What experts agree on is this: people in most countries rely on wheat for their diets, so wheat growing covers more arable land than does any other crop. In the United States alone, figures from the USDA show that in 2007, American farmers produced more than 2 billion bushels of wheat.

Why Wheat?

What makes wheat so coveted is its transformation into a delicious and nutritious end product, from cereals to flours for breadstuffs to pastas to certain alcohols. It's also a source of proteins, vitamins, and minerals.

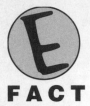

According to the Western Organization of Resource Councils, people in almost every country get at least 20 percent of their overall calories from wheat.

In its whole form, wheat is found as whole wheat kernels, or wheat berries, or as cracked wheat that is coarse, medium, or fine grained. What's confusing is that cracked wheat is commonly mistaken for bulgur—also known as bulghur or bulgar—a popular Middle Eastern wheat product made from steamed or parboiled, dried, and crushed wheat kernels. Cracked wheat comes from the whole wheat kernel that is broken into small, medium, or fine pieces. Both make fine pilafs and salads.

Not everyone can follow a wheat-based diet. Wheat contains the protein gluten, an element that helps bread rise but also causes negative immune responses in about 1 out of every 100 Americans, a condition know as celiac disease.

Other wheat varieties gaining in popularity are the less familiar—and ancient—wheats known as farro (*triticum dicoccum*) and its cousin, the European wheat spelt (*triticum speltum*), and the American-trademarked wheat known as Kamut. While relatively hard to find in supermarkets, whole-grain farro and spelt are available at health food markets. Almost indestructible, these firm grains do require soaking, but then can be boiled or sautéed for wholesome entrées.

Rice

Rice is grown almost everywhere in the world, and it is truly a beloved food for numerous reasons: it is plentiful, delicious, inexpensive, and very filling.

Rice is also nutritious, since it contains several vitamins and minerals, complex carbohydrates, and no fat. Because it still contains the bran, brown rice provides more nutrients and has a more complex, slightly nutty taste.

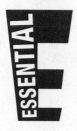

The Chinese value rice so much that when they greet each other, their salutation may be "Have you eaten your rice?" And when they go off to have a meal, they often say they are going to "eat rice," regardless of what is really on the menu.

Varieties of Rice

According to The Rice Association, at least 40,000 varieties of cultivated rice exist, though only a fraction of that number ever finds its way to the marketplace and to the cookpot. Rice is generally divided into three categories: long grain, medium grain, and short grain.

And within those categories, you'll find numerous varieties, from the long-grain fragrant basmati and jasmine rice preferred in India and parts of Asia to the regular unscented long-grain rice the Chinese and Americans cook. Medium- and short-grain rice tends to be moister and plumper—and the very short-grain rice used for sushi has a sticky quality that lets the grains cling together.

Because rice is very versatile, it can be processed into an "instant" rice; ground up for flour; steamed, stir-fried, baked, or sautéed; and even turned into wine and beer. Some Asians also shape rice to fit into a hollow bamboo tube for grilling, roll it into a ball for wrapping in a banana leaf, or form it into cakes as a garnish for a main dish. And the Japanese celebrate the New Year with a rice cake called *mochi*, made from cooked and pounded glutinous rice.

How to Cook Perfect Rice

For best results, and for the cleanest rice, you should rinse the grains under cold water until the water runs clear. Then comes the "how-to-cook" challenge. Asian cooks are so adept at cooking rice that many are able to judge the grains on their age and country of origin when deciding how much water to use. For that reason, the water-to-rice ratio varies anywhere from two parts water to one part rice to an even ratio of one to one. But a general rule of thumb is this: the "knuckle method" calls for pouring the rice into a pot, and filling it with cold water to one knuckle's height above the top of the rice. Do not add salt or butter. Cook the rice uncovered in boiling water for several minutes—or as some Asians say, until "dragon's eyes" (bubbles) appear on the surface—then reduce the heat to low and cover the pot. After ten or so minutes, the grains will be tender. Note that this refers to an Asian method of cooking long-grain white rice, their preferred grain; Western methods may differ. Brown rice requires more water and longer cooking. For detailed Western rice-cooking instructions, visit *www.usarice .com/consumer/prep.html*.

That's a fine, old-fashioned way to cook rice, but rice cookers make rice cooking just about foolproof. Just follow the manufacturer's directions. Of course, you won't need to puzzle over the rice's origin or age either.

Barley and Oats

Both barley and oats are ancient grains with outstanding pedigrees—that is, both have contributed beneficial nutrients to the human diet, from necessary complex carbohydrates to protein, minerals, and fiber. And both have played their part in the daily menu as the basis for breads, cooked cereal, soups, and, in the case of barley, beer.

About Barley

According to a study conducted by the Agricultural Research Service of the USDA, barley is a mega powerhouse filled with nutrients that aid in reducing the risk factors for developing type 2 diabetes and heart disease. But besides the study, health experts tout barley because it's also rich in soluble fiber, one of the elements that helps slow the absorption of sugar. Its insoluble fiber may also reduce the risk of some cancers. One study suggests that barley's insoluble fiber may even help prevent gallstones in women. Note that one cup of barley contains 13.6 grams of fiber.

Achieving good health is one reason to eat barley. Another is enjoying its versatility. When cooked, its chewy grains and nutty flavor enhance a variety of dishes, from soups, porridges, and stews to stuffings and pilafs. Barley is available in the market as either quick-cooking flakes or slower-cooking barley pearls. In health food stores, you can also find hulled, or whole grain, barley, which requires soaking and longer cooking times. For complete barley information, check out *www.barleyfoods.org*.

About Oats

Another of Mother Nature's wholesome and ancient grains, oats have not always found favor on the table. In ancient times, both the Greeks and the Romans spurned oats in favor of wheat. Englishmen once thought oats were fit only for horse feed; their Scottish compatriots, on the other hand, have long favored oats as a sustaining cereal; hence, the Scottish favorite— an old-fashioned breakfast of porridge oats.

When oats arrived in the New World, Americans grew it primarily as horse feed—that is, until two entrepreneurs developed a machine that could easily cut oat groats, or whole oats, into a steel-cut oatmeal for a palatable cereal. Today's mass-marketed morning oatmeal comes as quick-cook or instant cereals, flavored with assorted tastes, though the old-fashioned rolled oats are still available.

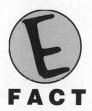

FACT

When research pinpointed oats—and oat bran—as a valuable agent for reducing blood cholesterol and cutting the risks of heart disease, oats became a fashionable mainstream breakfast cereal as well as an ingredient used in numerous other products, from beer to breads to cosmetics.

As you shop for oats, you may find a bewildering number of oat products, including whole oats, which require soaking and lengthy cooking for softening; oat bran, the oat grain's outer casing; steel-cut oats, or whole oats chopped into smaller pieces; rolled or old-fashioned oats, or oat groats that are steamed then rolled flat; quick-cooking oats, or groats cut into small pieces before steaming and flattening; and instant oats, highly processed groats that have been chopped, precooked, dried, and flattened. Whichever form you buy, remember that oatmeal contains a small amount of fat, so it tends to turn rancid more quickly than other cereals—store it in a cool, dark place.

Exotic Grains: Amaranth, Millet, and Quinoa

Among the multitudes of grains there are several that seldom see a Western cookpot, though they have places on menus elsewhere in the world. They may sound and even look exotic, but the canny vegetarian will make room in the kitchen pantry for them and make sure these grains find their way into recipes as often as possible. For like their more common kinfolk, these grains, too, are nutrient workhorses.

Amaranth

The amaranth plant's tiny tan seeds are nutritious and apparently were grown and eaten by the ancient Incas, Mayans, and Aztecs, the latter believing the seeds contained some potent magic that gave people power. Today, amaranth seeds are valued for their high protein content—especially the amino acid lysine—as well as their vitamins, minerals, and fiber. The leaves of the plants figure as a vegetable in some Latino countries. Amaranth cooks in a covered pot in about twenty minutes, with a ratio of one part amaranth to three parts water.

Millet

Bland millet seeds—golden, red, or white—are popular for their nutritional profile, particularly in Asia and Africa. A serving offers beneficial amounts of niacin, magnesium, and phosphorous, and millet offers a significant benefit in cutting down on the risk of heart disease and type 2 diabetes.

Like amaranth, millet cooks in water with a ratio of one part millet to three parts water. Cook covered for about twenty-five minutes.

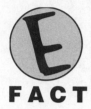

FACT

Quinoa seeds are naturally coated in a substance called saponin, a bitter-tasting compound that may cause intestinal upsets for some people. Saponin is easily removed by rubbing the seeds between your hands in water.

Quinoa

An ancient food favored by the Incas and other South American native peoples, quinoa (pronounced KEEN-wa) is not actually a cereal, grain, or grass, but is instead the seed of a leafy green vegetable. A source of complete amino acids, the word *quinoa* translates from the Quechua language as "the mother grain." Its value for the Incas came from its energy-sustaining properties, which some suggest allowed Incas to march or run for days on a handful of the seeds. Besides protein, quinoa also contains various minerals.

SERVES 4

400 calories
18g fat
45g carbohydrates
19g protein
840mg sodium
9g fiber

INGREDIENTS:

3 tablespoons vegetable oil

8 ounces firm tofu, cubed

3 cloves garlic, crushed and minced

1 onion, diced

1 tablespoon minced fresh ginger, or to taste

1 cup cubed winter squash, such as butternut or kabocha

1 cup shelled edamame

1 (8-ounce) can sliced bamboo shoots, drained

2 long, green chiles, thinly sliced

2 cups cooked short-grain brown rice, chilled

3 tablespoons soy sauce, or to taste

½ cup vegetable broth or water, as needed

Asian Stir-Fried Rice

When cooking tofu, you need to press out the excess water, otherwise it splatters in hot oil and doesn't brown well. To do this, slice a block of tofu in half and wrap the cut pieces in layers of paper towels, changing the towels for new sheets when these get soaked. Some cooks suggest weighting the blocks of tofu down to press out more water.

1. Heat the oil in a large wok or skillet over medium-high heat. Add and stir-fry the tofu, cooking it until it starts to brown. Remove it from the wok and set aside.

2. Add the garlic, onion, and ginger and stir-fry for about 1 minute. Add the squash and edamame and stir-fry about 2 minutes. Add the bamboo shoots, chiles, and rice, stirring well to combine. Add the soy sauce and cover the wok, cooking the mixture for about 5 minutes or until the squash becomes tender. During the cooking, check that the mixture does not get too dry and add vegetable broth as needed, stirring it in well. Serve hot.

Why Chill the Rice?

If you don't chill cooked rice for stir-frying, the grains clump together and become mushy; also it's likely they will absorb too much oil during the cooking. Besides, stir-frying is a great way to use up leftover rice. This recipe calls for short-grain brown rice, which is somewhat sticky, but it provides a delicious texture and flavor for this dish. Any leftover rice will work.

Apple, Quince, and Barley Tart

For convenience sake, use a ready-made piecrust just out of the freezer. This meal comes together quickly. Despite its sweetness, the dish makes a pleasant supper or brunch main course because the barley provides an earthy flavor counterpoint to the apple and jelly. A lisht, tart side salad makes the perfect accompaniment.

1. Preheat the oven to 350°F.

2. Combine the eggs and cheese in a large mixing bowl and stir in the barley, apple, quince, and dates. Mix together well and spoon the mixture into the piecrust. Spoon the apple jelly over top.

3. Bake for about 30 minutes or until the crust browns. Cool slightly before serving.

What Is Quince?

A favorite Mediterranean, Asian, and Hispanic fruit, the quince resembles a green-yellow apple, but its flesh is very firm and its flavor is tart. Quince is high in pectin and adds a thickening power to jams and jellies. Some folktales attribute healing powers to quince: it purportedly cures upset stomachs, among other ills.

SERVES 4 TO 6

370 calories
16g fat
49g carbohydrates
11g protein
190mg sodium
4g fiber

INGREDIENTS:
2 large eggs, lightly beaten
1 cup shredded Swiss cheese
2 cups cooked and cooled barley
1 firm cooking apple, cored and sliced
1 quince, peeled, cored, and sliced
½ cup chopped dates
1 (9-inch) deep-dish piecrust
3 tablespoons apple jelly

270 calories
4.5g fat
58g carbohydrates
6g protein
30mg sodium
11g fiber

INGREDIENTS:
¾ cup fine-grain bulgur
1¼ cups boiling water
2 bunches scallions, finely
  sliced
2 small cucumbers, preferably
  Kirby, diced
1 bunch mint, rinsed and finely
  chopped
1 bunch parsley, rinsed and
  finely chopped
½ cup chopped dates
½ cup raisins
1 tablespoon olive oil, or more
  to taste
1 tablespoon lemon juice, or
  more to taste
Salt to taste

Bulgur Salad

Unlike the classic Lebanese tabbouleh, this bulgur salad contains several unconventional ingredients, imparting a slightly sweet taste to the dish. Yet like the traditional tabbouleh, this contains ample chopped parsley—plus chopped mint—so that the dish looks more green than brown.

1. Soak the cracked wheat in the boiling water and let it absorb the liquid for about 20 minutes. After that time, if any water remains, drain it off so the grains are plump but dry.

2. Meanwhile, combine the remaining ingredients in a large bowl, tossing to combine well. Add the bulgur and toss together well. Set aside for about 1 hour so the flavors can mingle.

What Is Tabbouleh?
A popular Middle Eastern salad dish, tabbouleh traditionally contains much more chopped parsley than cracked wheat; the wheat is almost like an afterthought or a garnish. This should be accompanied by bread for sopping up the olive oil and lemon juice; a traditional tabbouleh probably has about ¼ cup olive oil as part of the dressing.

Quinoa-Blueberry Pancakes

Serve these nutritious and hearty pancakes with a soy "sausage" crumbles or links. Serve the pancakes with melted butter and maple or fruit syrup or honey.

1. Stir together the eggs, yogurt, and melted butter. Stir in the blueberries and quinoa. Fold in the flour, sugar, baking powder, baking soda, and salt and mix until just blended.

2. Spray a nonstick griddle or large skillet with nonstick cooking spray and heat the griddle over medium-low to medium heat. Drop the batter by large spoonfuls onto the heated griddle and cook until the bottoms turn golden. Flip the pancakes over, respraying the skillet as needed. Remove the pancakes from the skillet when both sides are golden and the centers are firm. Repeat with the remaining batter and serve immediately.

SERVES 4

390 calories
15g fat
54g carbohydrates
12g protein
740mg sodium
6g fiber

INGREDIENTS:

2 large eggs, well beaten
1 cup plain yogurt
3 tablespoons melted butter or soy margarine
1 cup fresh or frozen blueberries
1 cup cooked quinoa
1 to 1¼ cups white whole wheat flour
2 to 3 tablespoons sugar
2 teaspoons baking powder
1 teaspoon baking soda
½ teaspoon salt

SERVES 4

310 calories
15g fat
43g carbohydrates
8g protein
290mg sodium
7g fiber

INGREDIENTS:

3 tablespoons olive oil
1 onion, diced
4 cloves garlic, minced
1 red bell pepper, cut into strips
　　lengthwise
8 ounces sliced mushrooms
2 cups cooked barley flakes
½ cup vegetable broth or water
Salt and freshly ground black
　　pepper to taste
½ to ¾ cup crumbled feta
　　cheese for garnish
½ cup dried cranberries for
　　garnish

Barley Pilaf

Instead of using barley flakes, try using cooked hulled or pearl barley for a different texture. Instead of feta cheese, consider adding crumbled Gorgonzola cheese.

Heat the oil in a large skillet over medium heat and sauté the onion until golden, about 5 minutes. Add the garlic, pepper, mushrooms, and barley and sauté for about 5 minutes. Add the vegetable broth, salt, and pepper. When the liquid is absorbed, remove from the heat and garnish with the feta cheese and cranberries. Serve hot.

Oatmeal Pudding

If you like oatmeal—the old-fashioned, slow-cooking kind with plenty of flavor—you'll enjoy this grain treat for breakfast, lunch, or dinner. The best part is you can tailor this dish to suit your preferences for add-in fruits and for sweetness.

1. Preheat the oven to 350°F. Lightly butter a 2-quart baking dish.

2. Beat the eggs, ricotta cheese, brown sugar, and vanilla together. Stir in the milk and the oats and add the dried fruits. Spoon the mixture into the prepared dish.

3. Bake for 45 minutes to 1 hour or until the center is firm and the edges are golden. Eat hot or cold.

SERVES 4 TO 6

390 calories
11g fat
61g carbohydrates
12g protein
110mg sodium
4g fiber

INGREDIENTS:

2 large eggs
1 cup whole or skim milk ricotta cheese
½ cup packed brown sugar
1 teaspoon vanilla extract
2 cups whole or skim milk or water
1 cup old-fashioned rolled oats
½ cup raisins
½ cup dried cubed papaya
½ cup dried cubed pineapple
Maple syrup, applesauce, or fruit syrup as garnish

Pea Pulao

SERVES 2

380 calories
14g fat
56g carbohydrates
8g protein
520mg sodium
7g fiber

INGREDIENTS:
1 cup basmati rice
2 tablespoons vegetable oil
1 onion, peeled and thinly sliced
1 cardamom pod, split open
1-inch stick cinnamon
*½ teaspoon toasted cumin
     seeds*
1 cup peas, fresh or frozen
1 teaspoon salt
Crisp fried shallots for garnish
*Chopped hard-boiled eggs for
     garnish*

Crisp fried shallots are sold already prepared in Asian markets. But as with most foods, their flavor is sharper and cleaner if you fry them up fresh: simply slice shallots thinly and fry them in vegetable oil over medium to medium-low heat until they turn golden and crispy; keep an eye on them so they don't burn. Drain them on paper towels.

1. Soak the rice in cold water for at least half an hour, but one hour is preferable.

2. Meanwhile, heat the oil in a large skillet over medium heat and sauté the onion, cardamom, cinnamon, and cumin until the onion turns transparent and golden.

3. Drain the rice and add it to the skillet; sauté for about 3 minutes. Add the peas, salt, and 2 cups water and cover the skillet. Reduce the heat to low and cook the rice for about 15 minutes or until the rice is tender and the water has evaporated. Scoop the rice onto a serving platter and garnish it, as desired.

What Is Pulao?

Pilaf, or *pulao*, is a rice dish as ancient as India. It might have originated in Northern India, where it was customarily served to the Nabobs, or Persian princes. Many varieties of rice grow in India, but the best and the costliest is a fragrant, long-grained rice known as basmati, with its unforgettable, slightly sweet taste and delicate perfumed aroma. Fortunately, basmati rice is readily available in most supermarkets. Pilafs usually contain meat; this meatless version is perfect for vegetarians.

Wild Rice Stir-Fry with Snow Peas and Broccolini

With its delicate nutty flavor and sturdy texture, wild rice makes a delicious basis for any number of different add-in ingredients. Experiment!

1. Heat the oil in a large wok over medium to medium-high heat. Add the garlic, ginger, and wild rice and stir-fry for about 1 minute. Add the snow peas, broccolini, and water chestnuts and stir-fry for 3 to 4 minutes more, adding more oil if needed. Add the scallions, water-cornstarch slurry, hoisin sauce, and soy sauce. Reduce the heat to medium-low and cover the wok for 2 to 3 minutes.

2. Uncover the wok and stir the mixture for 2 more minutes or until the vegetables are tender. Spoon onto serving plates, garnish with cashews, and serve.

Wild Rice Is Not a Rice?

Despite its name, wild rice is *not* a rice but is instead a grass native to the Great Lakes region. Typically, the rice requires thorough rinsing and lengthy cooking to tenderize the grains. But some markets now sell pre-cooked wild rice in vacuum-sealed foil packets that requires only a few moments of reheating to ready it for the table.

SERVES 6

220 calories
8g fat
33g carbohydrates
6g protein
730mg sodium
4g fiber

INGREDIENTS:

3 tablespoons vegetable oil, or more if needed
4 cloves minced garlic
1 tablespoon minced fresh ginger
3 cups cooked wild rice
¼ pound snow peas, rinsed and trimmed
1 bunch broccolini, cooked until crisp-tender and chopped
1 (8-ounce) can water chestnuts, drained
1 bunch scallions, sliced
½ cup water mixed with 1 tablespoon cornstarch
5 tablespoons hoisin sauce
3 tablespoons soy sauce
Whole cashews for garnish

410 calories
15g fat
36g carbohydrates
46g protein
320mg sodium
12g fiber

INGREDIENTS:
*1 cup cooked and cooled quick-
  cooking barley flakes
1 cup soy "meat" crumbles
1 cup grated Cheddar cheese
2 eggs, lightly beaten
½ cup dried breadcrumbs
½ cup minced parsley
Seasoning salt to taste*

Barley Burgers on Rye Bread

*Serve these patties on thick-cut slices of buttered rye bread,
making a layered sandwich with sliced tomatoes and lettuce if
you wish. During cooking, these patties are delicate, so handle
them carefully; they will firm up once the cheese melts and the
patties cool slightly.*

1. Combine all the ingredients in a mixing bowl and stir well. Shape 4
   patties by scooping some of the mixture into a measuring cup about
   ¾ full. Pack them together firmly to prevent crumbling.

2. Spray a large skillet with nonstick cooking spray and heat over
   medium-low to medium heat. Carefully scoop the mixture into the
   hot skillet and repeat with the remaining mixture. Cook the patties
   until each are browned on the bottom; turn them over carefully to
   brown on the second side. Remove from the heat and let the patties
   cool slightly. Serve warm on bread.

Grain Salad in Pepper Halves

Many different cultures claim originating stuffed peppers as an entrée, and you can find delicious versions of it, especially in the Middle East. Often ground meat is the main filling, but this version uses the protein powerhouse, quinoa, as the main filling. Note that you may use a red, green, or yellow/orange pepper.

1. Stir together the quinoa, feta, pumpkin seeds, and mayonnaise. Gently spoon the quinoa mixture into the pepper halves, packing it down if necessary to prevent spilling. Set aside.

2. Line 2 individual serving plates with the lettuce. Place the pepper halves onto the lettuce, garnish each portion with cilantro leaves, and serve.

SERVES 2

340 calories
18g fat
38g carbohydrates
9g protein
240mg sodium
4g fiber

INGREDIENTS:
1 cup cooked quinoa or barley flakes
3 tablespoons crumbled feta
3 tablespoons toasted pumpkin seeds
2 tablespoons mayonnaise, or more as desired
1 large sweet bell pepper, split in half lengthwise and seeded
Red leaf lettuce for plating
Snipped cilantro leaves for garnish

CHAPTER 13

From the Vegetable Garden

In the words of the esteemed late American food writer, M. F. K. Fisher, "There are many ways to love a vegetable. The most sensible way is to love it well-treated" (*How to Cook a Wolf*). And probably the most sensible way to treat your vegetables well is to pick up your trowel and lovingly plant your own vegetable garden. Selecting your seeds, tilling the dirt, treating the plants organically, and letting Mother Nature do her share leads straight to vegetable love. What else can rival the taste sensations of eating just-picked vegetables?

Veggies: Growing Your Own

When you think about it, working the land is part of the great American heritage, and even for urban dwellers with no more growing space than containers on a balcony, tending plants satisfies the inner pioneer spirit. In the early 1980s, Marian Morash, in her iconic PBS show and its companion cookbook *The Victory Garden Cookbook*, reminded Americans about the joys of gardening as she demonstrated how beautiful and flavorful freshly raised and picked vegetables can be.

Whether it is frugality or the sustainable foods movement that has sparked greater consumer interest, vegetable gardening is increasingly popular. Featured in a June 2008 issue of the *Wall Street Journal*, the article "The Vegetable Patch" tells how Americans are increasingly digging up flowerbeds to plant vegetables instead, a trend that, according to the National Gardening Association, grows annually, with consumer spending for vegetable seedlings up by 21 percent since 2007—and the money spent on herb seedlings is rising even faster. Beating down big grocery bills is one incentive for this vegetable-gardening bonanza. But no one can argue with how easy it is to go pick your own vegetables and the pleasures of eating them moments later.

What to Grow

Seed catalogs, online gardeners' sites, and local nurseries and garden centers provide the seeds or seedlings, the soils and organic fertilizers, and the tools—and gardening advice—so you can start your own vegetable garden. Your only constraints are time, energy, and space. Other than that, and depending on climate and the seasons, you can select which vegetables you and your family love best. Most vegetables—and many fruits—are easy to grow at home or in a community garden. But be advised, once the crops come in, you may have more than you can eat or cook—so be selective on what and how much you plant. Also check with your local agricultural service or nursery to find out which vegetables grow best in your area.

Veggies in the Kitchen

As with supermarket or farmers' market vegetables, your home-grown vegetables need the same care in handling. Although you probably intend to cook them right away, you need to store extras carefully—see Chapter 7 for how to store vegetables. And if you have a bumper crop, you can freeze or can extras for eating later in the year. You can also turn extras into flavorful sauces for pastas or cook up a selection for homemade vegetable soups; eat some now and freeze the rest for later use.

Another option is to make your own vegetable stock, a handy flavor booster for any savory-dish recipe that calls for added liquids—such as cooking rice, barley, lentils, or other grains. Diced or cubed carrots, onions (with the skins on for added color), garlic, leeks, herbs, and celery are typical stock ingredients, but you can create your own recipe using your favorites, even adding vegetable parings. For a more intense flavor, sauté your vegetables in olive oil before combining them with water in the stockpot.

Onions and Garlic

Favorite flavor enhancers, onions, garlic, scallions, and leeks—members of the *alliaceae* family—have universal appeal and have found their way into the global cookpot—from Europe to Asia to Latin America and the United States. Some gardeners use these plants as ornamentals, but the good cook knows: when added to almost any savory dish, onions, garlic, and leeks make flavors sing.

Health Benefits

Besides adding flavor, onions, and particularly garlic, have long been touted as beneficial for your health, and their purported medicinal uses—such as reducing blood pressure, working as an antibiotic, fighting certain cancers, and cleansing the arteries, for example—date back to centuries before the Christian Era. Today, some people suggest garlic as a supplement to reduce cholesterol and clear clogged arteries, and recent research at the National Academy of Sciences shows that garlic-rich diets may protect against various cancers and heart disease.

Rich in chromium and vitamin C, onions also reportedly yield health benefits, including lowering blood sugar, reducing high blood pressure, and mitigating the pain of arthritis. Also, the cancer-fighting phytonutrients, such as the antioxidant quercitin found in onions, may aid in fighting colon, breast, and ovarian cancers, among others.

Onions

Onions come in many sizes and shapes, ranging from the small, white pearl onions to the round, red onions to the slightly flattened, golden-skinned Vidalia and the smaller Italian cippolini. These onions are "cured" so that the skin turns papery, protecting the onion interior from decay; these must be stored in cool, dry places, not in the refrigerator. The other stalk-like onions—leeks and scallions, for example—are always fresh, with white bulbs and long, green, leaves furled lengthwise; these fresh onions should be plastic-wrapped and refrigerated. For more information, visit *www .fruitsandveggiesmatter.gov/month/leeks.html.*

ALERT!

If you are among the many who cry when slicing onions, numerous folk remedies abound, and it's anyone's guess about which method really works. But you can try several of these tricks: partially freeze or chill the onions before slicing them; slice the onions under running water; wear glasses or goggles; breathe through your mouth, not your nose; and use a very sharp knife, slicing off the root end first where the chemicals are concentrated.

Garlic

Fresh heads of garlic are readily available in supermarkets, and for added convenience, many manufacturers now sell prepeeled garlic cloves, chopped garlic packed in oil, garlic pastes, garlic salt, and dried garlic flakes. But for the best flavors, it's hard to pass up the fresh heads in their papery coverings.

Be sure to select heads that are firm without any soft spots or green sprouts, both signs of garlic going bad. At home, store garlic in a cool, dry place, discarding any cloves that are beginning to soften. To cook with garlic, separate the cloves from the head pressing down on the whole head with your hand or with the flat side of a cleaver or other broad knife. Then peel the papery skins off each clove, and crush or mince the garlic as desired.

Culinary Herbs

Herbs add that seductive bit of flavor to your cooking, and that first bite of Aha! in your mouth. Unlike spices—which are gleaned from seeds, barks, and roots—herbs are fresh or dried leaves that impart a mild yet distinctive flavor to recipes.

Selecting the right herb or herbs for that burst of taste is a bit like sampling chocolates or coffee flavors, for in each case you are looking for the best fragrance and taste experience. When you are seasoning, start small, adding a little of a single herb at a time until you find the balance you want. Then play around with your seasonings, using herbs in various compatible combinations.

You should try to use fresh herbs whenever possible; dried herbs lose potency quickly and must be used sparingly. Dried herbs also produce a much more intense flavor because their natural oils have become concentrated. If you are using them dried, check the herbs before seasoning: if their aroma seems musty or their color has turned grayish, they are probably past their potency, and you should discard them.

Culinary herbs are easy to grow, but you should pick the leaves before the plants start to flower, for flowers are a sign that the leaves may be turning bitter. If your herb crop is too large for quick use, you can pick the leaves and stems, and dry them for later use.

The Parsleys

An essential herb, parsley in all its various guises—curly-leaf and flat-leaf—not only garnishes plates and a finished dish, it also add its own characteristic flavor that ranges from mildly pungent to earthy-soapy, as some describe cilantro. Besides its uses in the kitchen, according to some research from the University of Kentucky, parsley also may offer several health benefits: it is an antioxidant, and it also may help prevent or deter certain cancers.

Although it is botanically a member of the carrot family, cilantro, also known as Chinese parsley, is used much the same way as standard parsley: as a garnish and as a flavor booster. The leaves of the coriander plant, cilantro is a must-have seasoning in many Hispanic, Caribbean, Asian, and Indian dishes; many North American cooks, too, have come to appreciate its pungent-acidic-earthy taste. Of course, whole or ground coriander seeds are mainstays of many international kitchens.

The Basils

Considered by many as the king of herbs, basil in all its forms—from the richly scented Thai basils to the sweet basils such as lemon basil, cinnamon basil, and Genovese basil—is an annual that is easy to grow and fortunately, is available year round in most supermarkets; some varieties are classed as tender perennials. Beloved for its minty fragrance and flavor accent, the basils also contain essential oils that may figure in reducing inflammation, fighting certain bacteria, and even promoting heart health.

Tarragon, Dill, Oregano, and Thyme

Strongly flavored, these herbs play critical roles in seasoning savory dishes, but all should be used sparingly until you find your comfort level with their flavors. Tarragon, with its unmistakable minty taste, plays a key role in French cooking and is used often in herb blends. Dill, or dill weed, is a parsley relative. Its fresh feathery leaves highlight breads, salads, and cheese, but because its leaves are heat sensitive, dill should be added to hot dishes just before serving; its seeds are favored for pickling and in salad dressings. Hailing originally from the Mediterranean region, oregano is popular worldwide for its earthy aroma that accents every kind of ingredient. Thyme has a warm yet delicate taste that heightens the flavors of many vegetarian dishes.

The Mints

A many-splendored and many-faceted herb with a lively and complex flavor, mint in its many guises suits both sweet and savory dishes and mint makes an elegant addition to a variety of beverages, including Kentucky's famed mint julep. Most mints are easy-to-grow perennials and, with careful tending, spread prolifically.

Squashes: Summer and Winter Varieties

A member of the gourd family, the squash—both summer and winter varieties—are nutrient-dense vegetables that can grace the cookpot all year long. Most varieties are easy for home gardeners to raise, though the winter squash plants spread lavishly and require more land than the average suburban dweller may wish to dedicate to growing squash.

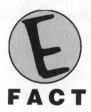

FACT

Both summer and winter squash offer certain health benefits that may make them good disease fighters: with their light- to deep-orange flesh, winter squash are rich in vitamin A, vitamin C, folate, and potassium. Summer squash contain respectable amounts of vitamin A, vitamin C, magnesium, potassium, and riboflavin.

Winter Squash

Best in late fall to early winter, the robust winter squash grows in numerous round to oval to pear shapes, with skin colors that range from white to orange to very dark green. Winter squashes include the buttercup, butternut, acorn, and pumpkin varieties.

Because their outer skin is hard, it is inedible, and you need to cut through it to reach the inner cavity, with its flesh, fibers, and seeds; you need to scrape out the fiber and seeds. You can bake these squashes whole and cut them up after baking, cut them into sections and cook the sections, or peel off the skin and cut up the flesh into chunks for adding to stews and soups or to roast for other dishes.

Summer Squash

Although most of these squashes are available throughout the year, they are vine-ripe and ready locally—in cooler climates—by early to midsummer.

Summer squashes include the light and darker yellow varieties, zucchini, pattypan, and crookneck.

Because each has an easy-to-slice skin and soft interior, the many summer squash varieties make fine additions to any type of dish, even breads and desserts in the case of zucchini, and they adapt themselves to many different cooking styles.

On the Stalk and from the Vine

Tomatoes, corn, asparagus, peas, peppers, cucumbers, green beans, and chiles: these assorted vegetables are so familiar in the kitchen that few cooks need an introduction. And most grow easily in a garden plot with enough room to accommodate their spreading vines and leafing stalks. Seeds and edible pods—from green beans to corn on the cob—are sweet when young and best if cooked straight from the garden or field. In the market, avoid any that look wrinkled or yellowing, which means they are old.

The summertime favorites—tomatoes, peppers, cucumbers, eggplants, and chiles—are basically available year round, but as any cook knows, their flavors reach their peak in the warm summer months. At home, most work well in a variety of recipes, making them ready nutrient sources.

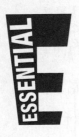

The heirloom tomato from the heritage varieties of yesteryear is the superstar of the tomato crop. Often asymmetrical and vividly colored—think purple, black, white, or yellow-striped green for a start—heirloom tomatoes often have intense tomatoey flavors that outshine the pallid supermarket types. If your market does not carry any, head to the nearest farmers' market in summertime, and take your pick!

Tomatoes

Perhaps one of the world's most popular vegetable—a gift to the kitchen from the fields of New World farmers—the tomato is not a vegetable at all but is really a fruit, a member of the nightshade family. Yet the tomato in its almost infinite number of sizes, shapes, and colors complements savory ingredients. It's also one of summertime's biggest hits, and although flavorful tomatoes are occasionally available throughout the year, their peak essence comes in mid- to late summer.

Tomatoes are a very rich source of the phytochemical lycopene, which research shows is a powerful antioxidant that may help protect against cancer. Tomatoes also contain ample amounts of vitamin C and assorted other nutrients, such as potassium and niacin.

Peppers

The sweet bell peppers have long been kitchen favorites, and probably thanks to the proliferation of Mexican and Asian foods, with their reliance on chili heat, the hot chiles have come into their own. At either end of the heat spectrum, the pepper makes a meal come alive: large peppers are easy to stuff, easy to roast and peel, easy to chop fresh in salads, and easy to sauté with one or many other ingredients. All you need do is watch for your favorite variety at the market, or as summertime wanes, explore the numerous kinds on sale at your farmers' market.

Hot peppers—the beloved chiles that perk up bland foods—are more readily available in a variety of fresh and canned forms. Perhaps the most familiar is Mexico's heat-bearing jalapeño and its red, smoked (or oven-dried) form, the chipotle, but increasingly you can locate the incendiary habanero and, from Thailand and Korea, the long and short chiles that cause their own sting. Just remember when handling hot chiles, wear rubber gloves and rinse your hands well after slicing them. If not, and you touch your skin or eyes, you will feel the burn.

But the best news is this: peppers are very easy to grow, even in small gardens. When the crop comes in, you'll have plentiful peppers, just for the picking. Note that many Asians enjoy eating the leaves of the hot peppers, stir-frying them with other greens or as a garnish for rice.

SERVES 6

330 calories
23g fat
17g carbohydrates
14g protein
230mg sodium
1g fiber

INGREDIENTS:

2 tablespoons olive oil
1 tablespoon minced garlic
About 2 cups coarsely chopped
*   peppers of your choice*
4 eggs, well beaten
1 cup milk
1 cup shredded Swiss cheese
1 to 2 teaspoons smoked
*   paprika*
Salt and freshly ground black
*   pepper to taste*
1 (9-inch) deep-dish piecrust

Peck of Peppers Tart

For this colorful entrée, mix and match the colors, sizes, and heat quotient of the peppers you select. If you don't want it too piquant, go easy on the hot chiles. Otherwise, live it up.

1. Preheat the oven to 350°F.

2. Heat the oil in a large skillet over medium heat and sauté the garlic. Add the peppers and sauté for 2 to 3 minutes.

3. Meanwhile, mix the eggs, milk, cheese, paprika, salt, and pepper together until well combined. Stir in the peppers and pour the mixture into the piecrust.

4. Bake the tart for 30 minutes or until the center is firm and the top browns. Serve hot.

Country Corn Cakes

If you have the room, corn is an easy-to-grow garden vegetable best when just picked off the stalk. Good for either breakfast or supper, these corn cakes may be served with melted butter and maple syrup, fruit syrup, or applesauce.

1. Combine the buttermilk, egg, and butter in a large mixing bowl. Stir in the grits, flour, corn kernels, black-eyed peas, baking powder, baking soda, salt, and pepper; the batter will be thick.

2. Heat about 2 tablespoons vegetable oil in a large skillet or on a griddle over medium to medium-low heat. When the surface is hot, spoon about ¾ cup of batter per cake onto the surface, and when the bottom has browned, carefully turn the cake over to cook the second side. Be sure the skillet does not overheat, or the cakes will burn. Repeat until all the batter is used up, adding more oil as needed. Serve hot.

About Black-Eyed Peas

If you live in the South, you know the tradition: eat black-eyed peas on New Year's Day to bring good luck for the rest of the year. But these delicious legumes, also known as "cow peas," should be enjoyed often. These "peas" (they are actually beans) are rich sources of calcium, potassium, protein, and vitamin A.

SERVES 4

440 calories
9g fat
77g carbohydrates
13g protein
760mg sodium
5g fiber

INGREDIENTS:

1 cup buttermilk
1 egg, lightly beaten
2 tablespoons melted butter
1 cup uncooked grits or coarse cornmeal
1 cup all-purpose flour
1 cup corn kernels, preferably fresh
1 cup cooked black-eyed peas
1 tablespoon baking powder
1 teaspoon baking soda
Salt and freshly ground black pepper to taste
Vegetable oil for pan-frying

SERVES 2

570 calories
18g fat
73g carbohydrates
28g protein
1,130mg sodium
13g fiber

INGREDIENTS:

1 tablespoon vegetable oil
1 cup diced tomatoes
½ cup chopped onions
1 (9-ounce) package soy "meatballs"
½ cup chopped fresh cilantro
2 tablespoons sweet mango chutney
1 tablespoon Indian curry powder
1 teaspoon ground turmeric
Salt to taste
1 cup plain yogurt
2 large pita loaves, softened

Curried Meatballs in Pita

For a spicier filling, use hot mango chutney instead of the sweet and add 1 or 2 diced green chiles to the meatball mixture. If you can find them, use the Greek-style pita loaves, which are extra-large but require wrapping as these loaves don't slit open for an inner pocket.

1. Heat the oil in a large skillet over medium heat and sauté the tomatoes and onion until softened. Meanwhile, cut the "meatballs" in half and add them to the skillet, stirring well and cooking until they are heated through. Stir in the cilantro, chutney, curry powder, turmeric, and salt. Cook about 2 minutes more and stir in the yogurt. Cook 2 to 3 minutes more and set aside.

2. Spoon the mixture evenly into the pita pockets; alternatively, wrap the "meatballs" up in the pita, tucking one end up to prevent dripping.

Stir-Fried Green Beans with Asian Eggplant, Garlic, and Fried Tofu

This stir-fry works well as a topping over steamed brown rice.

1. Mix the soy sauce, cornstarch, sugar, sesame oil, and water together and set aside.

2. Heat the oil in a large wok or skillet over medium-high heat. Add the garlic and ginger and stir-fry for 30 seconds. Add the beans, eggplants, tofu, and scallions and stir-fry for 2 to 3 minutes; if the mixture seems too dry, add a little water.

3. Stir in the soy sauce mixture and stir to coat all the vegetables. Keep stirring for about 2 more minutes or until the vegetables are crisp-tender. Remove from the heat and serve.

About Asian Eggplants

The general eggplant category known as Asian eggplant includes the long, slender, pale purple variety used in Chinese cooking and the slightly plumper and darker purple ones favored in Japan. Thais also favor a small, round, green or white eggplant that resembles plump golf balls or very small green ones that resemble peas. Look for these eggplants in well-stocked supermarkets or in Asian groceries.

SERVES 4

430 calories
26g fat
39g carbohydrates
17g protein
520mg sodium
13g fiber

INGREDIENTS:

2 tablespoons soy sauce, or more to taste
1 tablespoon cornstarch
1 tablespoon sugar
2 teaspoons toasted sesame oil
1 cup water
3 tablespoons vegetable oil
1 tablespoon minced garlic
1 tablespoon minced ginger
1 pound green beans, trimmed
1 Chinese or Japanese eggplant, cut into 2-inch-long pieces
3 Thai eggplants, quartered
1 (9-ounce) package fried tofu, cut into small pieces
1 bunch scallions, trimmed

Turkish-Style Stuffed Pepper

SERVES 1

470 calories
4g fat
83g carbohydrates
39g protein
35mg sodium
18g fiber

INGREDIENTS:

1 large red bell pepper
Olive oil for rubbing
½ cup cooked brown rice
¼ cup soy "meat" crumbles
2 tablespoons raisins
2 tablespoons chopped dried apricots
2 tablespoons chopped fresh mint
2 tablespoons chopped parsley
2 tablespoons plain yogurt

You can easily double or triple this recipe to serve more people, but it's so easy to prepare, it's fine just for one. For added texture, add a tablespoon or two of toasted pine nuts.

1. Preheat the oven to 400°F.

2. Cut the top off the pepper and clean out the seeds and membranes. Rub the pepper inside and out with the olive oil.

3. Combine the rice with the soy "meat," raisins, apricots, mint, parsley, and yogurt. Carefully spoon the mixture into the hollow pepper. Prop the pepper upright in a baking dish.

4. Bake the pepper for 30 minutes or until the pepper is tender. Serve.

Tomato Pie with Mozzarella and Italian "Sausage"

This pie shows off summer's bounty by pairing farm-fresh tomatoes with parsley, basil, and mozzarella cheese—summertime's perfect quartet.

1. Preheat the oven to 350°F.

2. Combine the eggs, mozzarella cheese, and milk in a large bowl, beating to mix well. Stir in the parsley, basil, garlic, and Parmesan cheese.

3. Layer the "sausage" slices on the bottom of the pie shell, overlapping the pieces as needed. Layer the tomato slices on top and gently pour in the cheese mixture, making sure it flows beneath the tomatoes. Top the filling with the slices of mozzarella cheese.

4. Bake for about 25 minutes or until the top browns and the cheese mixture is firm. Cool slightly before slicing.

SERVES 4 TO 6

360 calories
23g fat
19g carbohydrates
19g protein
400mg sodium
2g fiber

INGREDIENTS:

2 large eggs, lightly beaten
1 cup shredded mozzarella cheese
½ cup whole milk
1 cup chopped parsley
½ cup chopped fresh basil, or to taste
1 tablespoon minced garlic
1 tablespoon grated Parmesan cheese
1 Italian-seasoned soy "sausage," thinly sliced
1 (9-inch) unbaked deep-dish pie shell
3 to 4 large ripe tomatoes, thinly sliced widthwise
6 thin slices mozzarella cheese

Roasted Asparagus with Mixed Summer Squashes and Peppers

SERVES 4

240 calories
15g fat
23g carbohydrates
6g protein
10mg sodium
6g fiber

INGREDIENTS:

¼ cup olive oil
3 tablespoons balsamic vinegar
1 tablespoon minced garlic
1 pound asparagus, stem ends trimmed
1 pound mixed summer squashes, thinly sliced
1 pound mini sweet peppers, stemmed and sliced in half lengthwise
2 to 3 hot peppers, or to taste, chopped
Seasoning salt to taste

Don't skip this warm-weather dish if you cannot find the mini sweet peppers; simply substitute red, yellow, or green bell peppers.

1. Preheat the oven to 400°F.

2. Mix the olive oil, balsamic vinegar, and garlic together and set aside.

3. Place the vegetables into a large roasting pan, mixing them together so the flavors will mingle. Pour the olive oil mixture over top, lifting and gently mixing the vegetables so they are all coated with oil. Sprinkle the vegetables with seasoning salt.

4. Roast the vegetables uncovered for about 45 minutes or until they begin to darken; stir occasionally. Serve hot.

Heirloom Tomato Sandwich

Select a rustic-peasanty round loaf, such as a sourdough, and cut thick slices from the center for a full-sized sandwich. To kick this up a notch, use fresh mozzarella, which you should find in a specialty cheese shop or in the imported cheeses section of well-stocked supermarkets.

1. Drizzle the olive oil on 1 slice of bread.

2. Mix together the garlic and mayonnaise and spread the mixture on the other slice.

3. Cover this slice with basil leaves. Top the leaves with the tomato and the mozzarella slices, layering the slices if necessary. Sprinkle the slices with salt and pepper and close the sandwich.

SERVES 1

680 calories
29g fat
76g carbohydrates
25g protein
1,190mg sodium
6g fiber

INGREDIENTS:

1 teaspoon extra-virgin olive oil, or more as desired

2 thick slices bread, preferably sourdough

1 teaspoon minced garlic

2 teaspoons mayonnaise, or more as desired

Fresh basil leaves

1 large heirloom tomato, thinly sliced

2 thin slices fresh mozzarella cheese

Salt and freshly ground black pepper to taste

Chilaquiles with Green Sauce and Soy "Meat"

SERVES 6

770 calories
43g fat
64g carbohydrates
40g protein
1,050mg sodium
14g fiber

INGREDIENTS:

2 tablespoons vegetable oil
4 cloves garlic
4 tomatillos, diced
1 onion, chopped
1 cup chopped sweet red pepper
1 (15½-ounce) can pinto beans, drained and rinsed
3 cups shredded pepper jack or Monterey Jack cheese
2 cups salsa, hot or mild
1 cup soy "meat" crumbles
1 teaspoon crushed oregano
1 teaspoon ground cumin
4 cups crushed tortilla chips
Chopped fresh cilantro for garnish
Chopped jalapeños for garnish, optional

This classic dish was created as a way to use up stale corn tortillas, or so the story goes, and practically every household surely has its own version. But there's no need to wait for corn tortillas to dry out; today's taco chips make a fine base for this easy-to-make dish. If you want to add even more heartiness, you can top each serving with a poached egg.

1. Preheat the oven to 350°F. Lightly butter a 3-quart baking dish.

2. Heat the vegetable oil in a large skillet over medium heat and sauté the garlic, tomatillos, onion, and red pepper until the vegetables soften, about 5 minutes. Add the beans, stirring well.

3. Meanwhile, in a large bowl, combine the shredded cheese, the salsa, the soy "meat," the oregano, and the cumin, mixing well. Line the bottom of the baking dish with 2 cups of the crushed chips. Combine the tomatillo mixture with the cheese mixture and pour into the prepared dish. Top the mixture with the remaining 2 cups of chips, pushing them down into the mixture.

4. Bake for 20 minutes or until the cheese is bubbly. Garnish with fresh cilantro and chopped jalapeños if desired.

What Are Tomatillos?

A small, green cousin of the tomato, a tomatillo is covered with a papery husk, which must be removed before cooking. Tomatillos with their slightly tart flavor are the foundation of green salsas.

English Garden Pea Soup

Pair this soup with a salad and fine artisan bread for a hearty and satisfying meal.

1. Heat the olive oil in a saucepan over medium heat and sauté the garlic and leek for 3 to 4 minutes.

2. Spoon this mixture into a blender or food processor. Add the peas, white wine, yogurt, and heavy cream if using. Purée until smooth. Season with salt and pepper. Pour into soup bowls and garnish as desired.

Rinsing Leeks

Because leeks are raised in mounds of sand, the grains of which seem to trickle freely between its tightly furled leaves in the stalk, leeks are notoriously gritty and require a thorough rinsing in cold water. One way to get rid of the sand is to slice from just above the root end (leave the root intact for this) and, using a very sharp knife, slit the leek in half lengthwise. Then swish the leek and its separated leaves through a sink of water. When the sand is gone, slice off the root and use.

SERVES 2

380 calories
16g fat
31g carbohydrates
10g protein
40mg sodium
8g fiber

INGREDIENTS:

1 tablespoon olive oil
2 cloves garlic, thinly sliced
1 leek, thinly sliced
2 cups garden peas
1 cup white wine
3 tablespoons plain yogurt
3 tablespoons heavy cream, optional
Salt and freshly ground black pepper to taste
Snipped chives for garnish
Garlic croutons for garnish
Soy bacon for garnish
Tarragon leaves for garnish

CHAPTER 14

Fruits and More Fruits

These sweet—and, sometimes, not-so-sweet—crops span the color chart from white to purple-black and all the rainbow hues in between. Every country grows one or another variety, every culture has its way with fruit, and every mealtime can get a lift with at least one serving.

14

The Basics of Fruits

In the kitchen, ripe fruits of any classification can come to the rescue morning, noon, and night—and in between. Fruits can stand alone and be enjoyed raw, with maybe a drizzle of honey, a slice of cheese, or a sprinkling of rum as flavor accents. On the other hand, many fruits cook up well in syrups, pies, cakes, jams, pancakes, waffles, custards, soufflés, ice creams, and puddings, and they can accent savory entrées with just a hint of sweetness to tempt the palate: plantains with black beans is one such example.

Fortunately, astute growers and vigilant green consumer groups have reignited the collective passion for the fruits of yesteryear, from the freeform colorful heirloom tomatoes to the desirable heirloom apples. Thanks to the efforts of several national groups, you, too—provided you have the space—can grow the same full-flavored varieties of apples, peaches, melons, paw paws, and tomatoes, plus others, that pleased generations past. Your growing such heirloom varieties has a double benefit: your eating pleasure and your preserving plant diversity. For more information, visit *www.seedsavers .org.*

Keys to a Healthy Diet

As with their vegetable cousins, fruits are healthful props for the modern diet. As the USDA points out, fruit—and vegetable—consumption may lower the risk factors for several chronic diseases, such as heart disease, type 2 diabetes, certain cancers, development of kidney stones, and, of course, obesity.

The USDA further details those nutrients in most fruits that act as health-promoting agents: potassium, in bananas, cantaloupe, and orange juice, for example, for its possibly normalizing blood pressure; vitamin C for tissue growth and repair; folate, for red blood cell formation; and that all-important fiber, for keeping the intestines functioning properly and for possibly reducing levels of blood cholesterol.

Experts from the Harvard School of Public Health say you should eat about two cups of fruit a day to promote, among other health benefits, better eyesight. Even the popular press has jumped on the "eat fruits" bandwagon by glorifying the benefits of such summer delicacies as blueberries, often touted for their ability to reduce the risk of certain cancers, to lower blood pressure, to fight infections, and, best of all, to keep minds sharp. Another fruit celebrity is cranberries, for their ability to fight urinary tract infections, as cited by the Cranberry Institute. And, of course, who hasn't heard the nursery jingle about eating daily apples to keep doctors away?

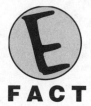

FACT

From the CDC, you'll read about how those who insert more fruit (and vegetable) servings per day into their diet are less likely to develop certain chronic diseases, confirming what others say. Its website, *www .fruitsandveggiesmatter.gov/benefits/index.html*, also charts which fruits contain which nutrients and celebrates the fruit of the month.

Fruits in the Kitchen

If you are trying to up your fruit intake, you might want to select precut fruits as time savers; you should buy seasonal fruits, which will cost less; and you should stock up on dried, frozen, or canned fruits (packed in juice, not syrup) so you'll have some at the ready. While you must refrigerate cut-up fruits, most whole fruits will last a day or so at room temperature—in either case, buy only what you can consume in a few days' time to prevent tossing out spoiled fruit later on. And for the best health benefits, select different fruit varieties, as each variety has different nutrients.

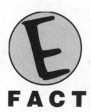

FACT

In its MyPyramid section on what counts as a serving of fruit, the USDA estimates that one cup of fruit or 100 percent fruit juice or a half cup of dried fruit counts as a one-cup serving. To envision what constitutes a serving, refer to this handy chart: *www.fruitsandveggiesmatter.gov/what/ index.html*.

Safe Fruit Handling

As with all fresh produce, fruits need a good rinsing to remove both farm dirt and invisible microorganisms before you plan to eat them. For fragile berries, a gentle spraying should do the trick without bruising them.

Firm fruits should be washed in warm—not hot—water. Even fruits whose skin you peel away should be gently rinsed.

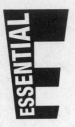

Note that fruitarians believe the only road to optimal health is by eating raw fruits and nuts exclusively. For more information, visit *www.fruitarian .com*.

The Citrus Connection

Probably everyone has seen the various television commercials for Florida orange juice, and maybe in the minds of many consumers, oranges are the only viable citrus fruits. Not so. According to a report issued by the United Nations Conference on Trade and Development, citrus fruits run the gamut from darling clementines that hit the market in fall and winter to pomelos in the winter to lemons, limes, and grapefruits, available pretty much the whole year. But oranges account for 70 percent of citrus crops grown in various countries.

As with various other members of the food world, citrus fruits may have first been picked in Southeast Asia, and they have been delighting the human palate probably since 4,000 B.C.

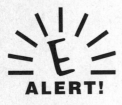

According to the USDA's MyPyramid, all fruits count, whether they are fresh, canned, cooked, dried, or juiced. But, warn the experts, 100 percent fruit juices don't contain the body's needed fiber, and "fruit-flavored" drinks rarely contain any fruit.

Citrus and Health

As a potent source of vitamin C in the form of ascorbic acid, citrus fruits have taken their place at the table, but you should know what other nutrients they offer: potassium, folate, calcium, thiamin, and various phytochemicals.

Besides, they are rich in fiber and in energy-producing carbs and contain no fat or cholesterol, a plus for dieters.

Because of their many health-conferring benefits, citrus fruits should be a dietary staple of people who are elderly, smoke, drink, have burns and/or are fighting infections.

Apples, Peaches, Plums, Pears, and More

The apple has been a longtime American favorite, and indeed, according to some apple experts, back in the early 1900s, an inventory listed at least 17,000 varieties worldwide. Today, probably only 2,000 to 3,000 apple varieties remain—which is why such organizations such as the Old-Time Apple Growers Association in central Virginia work to preserve heirloom varieties.

Peaches, of course, strike a happy chord with many people, both here and abroad. It's a joyous fruit, often talked about in terms of positive associations and life being wonderful. Perhaps its folklore is what links it to these positive thoughts: the Chinese have associated the peach with longevity. Available fresh in peak summer season, peaches also come canned and frozen. Its varieties include the freestone, the clingstone, and the semi-freestones. Perhaps the most intriguing peach is the doughnut-shaped one called the "doughnut" peach. The peach's nearest kin, the nectarine, is often thought of as a cross between a plum and a peach; in fact, the nectarine is a natural fruit with nearly 100 different varieties of freestone and clingstone fruits.

Related to peaches and nectarines, the plum apparently grew first in China before it began its global voyage. Although there are about 100 varieties, only 20 or so are readily sold in the marketplace from May through October. Plums also cook up well. It's worth noting that plums are recognized as a cure for constipation; the stimulating substance resides in the skin, so you may want to peel your plums first if need be.

A relative of the apple, the pear has often been reckoned as a gift from the gods, as the Greek writer Homer once described them. It is the honey-sweet flavor of its juicy flesh that makes this such a desirable fruit. Of the 3,000 or so varieties, perhaps the most notable ones are the Bartletts, red and green Anjous, and the Comice.

For more information about selecting, cleaning, and storing these popular fruits, go to *www.fruitsandveggiesmatter.gov/month*.

Going Bananas and Other Tropical Treats

By their nature and by their very definition, tropical fruits only flourish in parts of the world that maintain a constant temperate-to-hot climate year round. Numerous fruits fall within this category, from the very familiar bananas, pineapples, and avocados to the very unfamiliar mangosteens, star fruit, and custard apples. Fortunately for the passionate cook, such natural beauties as pomelos (which look like oversized grapefruit but have a sweeter character), yellow mangoes, and papayas—even the pungent durian from Southeast Asia—are now more readily available in well-stocked markets once they come in season.

Health Benefits

Most sources can describe the nutrient profiles of the commonplace fruits, but, according to a University of Florida document from the Institute of Food and Agricultural Sciences issued in September 2007, not much research has been done on the tropicals.

Reams of facts and legions of followers, however, have documented all aspects of the banana, the one tropical fruit that almost every American knows, if not adores. Portable for the lunchbox, sliceable for the breakfast cereal, and adaptable for the baking pan or the ice cream maker, the banana offers plenty under the skin: vitamins B_6 and C and the mineral potassium. Besides, a medium-size banana packs in only 110 calories, not bad for such a sweet treat. No wonder, as the Chiquita corporation has tracked, the typical American eats about twenty-seven pounds of bananas each year.

Berries, Cherries, and Grapes

Berries, cherries, and grapes are immensely popular additions to the table. While berries are the hallmark of warm-weather eating, thanks to technology and flash freezing, you can put berries in recipes all year round. Grapes, too, are readily available despite the season. A particularly sweet variety known as the muscadine shows up in late summer to early fall.

Good cooked or raw, berry varieties include the familiar blueberry, blackberry, strawberry, and raspberry, but plenty of others make their way to the marketplace. Also keep a look out for gooseberries, lingonberries, and currants.

Known as "stone fruits," cherries belong to the same family as berries and grapes and come in either sweet or sour types. Everyone knows the dark sweet Bing cherry, but the sweeter Rainier cherry is gaining in popularity.

Health Benefits

Media reports about blueberries as nuggets of health-containing phytochemicals are right: according to the USDA, researchers have identified compounds in blueberries—and in cranberries—that may protect against the blood vessel diseases.

Cherries contain some vitamins and minerals and no fat, cholesterol, or sodium. Sour cherries are richer in vitamin C than their sweeter relatives.

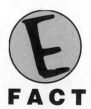

FACT

Members of the berry family, grapes help relax people, but they also work hard at combating several diseases, including certain cancers; slowing the effects of aging; and supporting heart health. To learn more, go to *www.tablegrape.com/phytonutrients.html*.

Melons

Members of the same botanical gourd family as squash and cucumbers, the melon dates back centuries to its first pickings in the Middle East, where in ancient times, the populace delighted in the juicy appeal of cantaloupes and muskmelons.

Today, what most people may not know is that melon varieties seem endless. You may be the most familiar with summer's honeydews, cantaloupes, and watermelons. But elsewhere, people slice into such melon selections as the Christmas, Sharlyn, canary, Sicilian, and Russian melon.

While the delicate and juicy flesh of the melon does not generally work well in baked goods, it does stand up well on its own or blended into power drinks.

According to the CDC, melons in general contain ample amounts of vitamin C and potassium. Besides, melons are also generally low in calorie, making them great choices for people watching their weight.

Banana-Pineapple-Yogurt Frosty

For a winning taste, look for a fruit yogurt made from one or a combination of tropical fruits. This liquidy mixture could be eaten with a spoon if allowed to freeze almost completely.

Combine all the ingredients in the container of a blender and process until smooth. Pour the mixture into a suitable container and chill in the freezer for about ½ hour or until ice forms around the edges of the container. Stir again and serve.

SERVES 2

350 calories
3.5g fat
69g carbohydrates
11g protein
125mg sodium
4g fiber

INGREDIENTS:

1½ cups nonfat milk or soymilk
1 (6-ounce) container nonfat
    tropical fruit yogurt
2 ripe bananas
1 cup well-drained crushed
    pineapple
2 teaspoons vanilla extract
2 teaspoons sugar, or to taste
Sprinkle ground nutmeg

310 calories
10g fat
50g carbohydrates
5g protein
75mg sodium
2g fiber

INGREDIENTS:
3 tablespoons cornstarch
2 cups almond-flavored soymilk
2 eggs yolks
½ cup sugar
2 teaspoons almond extract
1 teaspoon vanilla extract
Pinch salt
2 tablespoons butter
1 cup blueberries
1 cup sliced strawberries

Almond Cornstarch Fruit Pudding

An old-fashioned cornstarch pudding, this smooth and creamy mixture forms a soothing backdrop to the assertive fruit flavors. A cook's tip: before adding cornstarch to a liquid, always mix cornstarch first with a little liquid to make a paste. And don't whisk the cornstarch too vigorously because that causes it to break down so it won't thicken properly. Instead, stir it slowly with a wooden spoon.

1. Combine the cornstarch with 3 tablespoons soymilk, then combine this mixture with egg yolks and sugar in a mixing bowl. Stir in ½ cup soymilk to make a paste.

2. Heat the remaining soymilk in a large saucepan over medium-low to medium heat and, stirring gently, slowly pour in the cornstarch mixture. Increase the heat to medium-high and bring the mixture to a boil. Immediately reduce the heat to medium-low and, stirring gently, add the almond and vanilla extracts and the salt and butter.

3. Meanwhile, put the fruit into a 2-quart serving bowl. When the pudding mixture is thickened slightly, pour it over the fruit. Let the pudding cool slightly before serving or chill and serve cold.

Nectarine-Cherry Tart with Oat Crumble Topping

These ingredients come together to yield an old-fashioned taste treat. Instead of heavy cream, you may want to substitute vanilla ice cream.

1. Preheat the oven to 350°F.

2. Toss the nectarine slices and cherries together, then add ½ cup brown sugar and tapioca. When this mixture is well combined, add the butter and vanilla extract. Spoon the mixture into the piecrust.

3. To make the topping, combine the oats, pecan pieces, ½ cup brown sugar, flour, and butter and mix well until the topping is crumbly. Sprinkle over the filling and press down.

4. Bake until the crust and topping are brown, about 30 minutes. Serve warm and drizzle each slice with heavy cream, if using.

SERVES 4 TO 6

640 calories
33g fat
80g carbohydrates
10g protein
150mg sodium
5g fiber

INGREDIENTS:

2 large ripe nectarines, unpeeled and thinly sliced
2 cups fresh or frozen pitted cherries
½ cup firmly packed brown sugar
3 tablespoon instant tapioca
1 tablespoon firm butter, diced
1 teaspoon vanilla extract
1 (9-inch) deep-dish piecrust
1 cup old-fashioned rolled oats
1 cup toasted walnut pieces
½ cup brown sugar
3 tablespoons flour
¼ cup butter
Heavy cream for topping, optional

SERVES 6

610 calories
31g fat
78g carbohydrates
9g protein
330mg sodium
4g fiber

INGREDIENTS:
*1 (14-ounce) can condensed
    milk*
¾ cup lime juice
*1 pint fresh kumquats, stemmed
    and chopped*
*1 prepared 9-inch graham
    cracker crust*
1 cup heavy cream
2 tablespoons sugar

Kumquat Pie

A topping of sweetened whipped cream helps to glamorize this pie, but if you prefer, you can use a cup of sour cream spread over top before serving. Kumquats tend to be tart, however.

1. Combine the condensed milk with the lime juice, mixing together well. Fold in the kumquats and spoon the mixture into the crust. Refrigerate for at least 6 hours or overnight, or until the filling is firm.

2. Before serving, using chilled beaters, whip the cream until it begins to thicken and slowly stream in the sugar. When the mixture is thick, spread it evenly over the pie and serve.

What Are Kumquats?
A small, oval citrus fruit, the kumquat resembles a small orange—indeed, apparently its name translates as "gold orange" from Cantonese. Less sweet than an orange and less sour than a lemon, it is often preserved in sugar syrup. But the fresh kumquat is delicious, if a bit tart, eaten raw.

Mango Soup

Sinfully rich and deliciously spicy, this soup makes a perfect beginning for an exotic main course. If you want to cut calories, use light coconut milk and plain nonfat yogurt.

1. Combine the mango and mango nectar in a food processor or blender and purée for 30 seconds. Add the coconut milk, sour cream, lime juice, curry powder, and sugar. Process until smooth. Chill.

2. To serve, spoon the soup into individual bowls and arrange a circle of jalapeño slices in the middle of the bowl if using. Garnish the soup with julienned mint leaves.

SERVES 4

240 calories
18g fat
22g carbohydrates
3g protein
25mg sodium
3g fiber

INGREDIENTS:

2 cups mango cubes, preferably fresh
1½ cups mango nectar
1 cup coconut milk
½ cup sour cream
3 tablespoons fresh lime juice
1 teaspoon curry powder
Sugar to taste
2 jalapeños, thinly sliced, for garnish, optional
Julienned mint leaves for garnish

SERVES 4

180 calories
10g fat
19g carbohydrates
7g protein
510mg sodium
4g fiber

INGREDIENTS:
½ pound shredded green papaya
2 teaspoons minced garlic
5 to 6 fresh green chiles, thinly
   sliced
1 large ripe tomato, sliced
½ cup roasted peanuts
1 to 2 tablespoons lime juice
1 to 2 tablespoons soy sauce
Sugar to taste

Green Papaya Salad

This popular salad is a staple in Northern Thailand, where it is called som tam, *and in other parts of Thailand and in Laos, but its popularity has spread to this country, where diners can find it on many Thai restaurant menus. The traditional version uses fish sauce instead of soy sauce.*

Combine all the ingredients in a large mortar or mixing bowl and, using a pestle or sturdy wooden spoon, pound the ingredients together, tossing them to mix well.

What Is Green Papaya?
Generally considered a healthful fruit filled with several vitamins and containing the enzyme papain, the ripe orange papaya makes delicious eating on its own; its green, or unripened, counterparts are frequently used in Thai cooking. When shredded or cut up, the green papaya is used in curries or salads. Shredded green papaya is readily available in vegetable cases at Asian grocers, saving you the trouble of peeling and hand-grating the fruit.

Apple, Quince, and Goat Cheese Cake with Guava Paste

What makes this cake so delightful is that it whips up in minutes, and while it bakes, you can prepare other parts of the meal or read a book. You can vary the fruit to suit the season, omitting the brown sugar with very sweet fruit—and for the most delicious results, serve the cake at room temperature topped with plenty of ice cream.

1. Preheat the oven to 375°F. Butter and flour a deep 9-inch cake pan.

2. Put the first 4 ingredients in the food processor and pulse 2 or 3 times. Add the vanilla extract, flour, baking powder, and salt and pulse for 30 seconds or until smooth. Scrape into the prepared pan. Combine the apple and quince and toss with the brown sugar. Top the batter with the apple-quince mixture.

3. Bake for 40 minutes and place the goat cheese slices on top of the cake. Bake another 10 minutes or until a toothpick inserted in the center comes out clean. Remove from the oven, and cool completely. To serve, slice desired amounts of guava paste and garnish each serving with it.

What Is Guava Paste?

Made from guava pulp, pectin, and sugar, for commercial purposes the paste is formed into a rectangular block, wrapped and boxed, and sold at Hispanic markets and some supermarkets. It's a popular sweet at many Latino meals, served with bland cheese or used as a filling in pastries. It's also good sliced and eaten on hot toast in the morning.

SERVES 4 TO 6

360 calories
24g fat
27g carbohydrates
11g protein
170mg sodium
4g fiber

INGREDIENTS:
¼ pound (1 stick) unsalted butter
1 teaspoon lemon extract
1 teaspoon grated lemon zest
2 large eggs
1 teaspoon vanilla extract
1 cup white whole wheat or all-purpose flour
1 teaspoon baking powder
Pinch salt
1 apple, unpeeled and diced
1 quince, diced
2 tablespoons brown sugar
4 ounces goat cheese, sliced
Sliced guava paste, as desired
Ice cream, as desired

SERVES 9

370 calories
19g fat
46g carbohydrates
5g protein
200mg sodium
3g fiber

INGREDIENTS:

½ cup (1 stick) unsalted butter
8 ounces white chocolate
¾ cup firmly packed light brown
    sugar
1 egg, lightly beaten
1 cup white whole wheat flour
1 teaspoon baking powder
1 teaspoon salt
⅓ cup dried blueberries, or
    more as desired
⅓ cup dried cranberries or dried
    cherries, or more as desired

Fruited Blondies

*Typically, brownies are just chocolate with nuts sometimes
mixed into the batter. But this takes the fudgie brownie to a
different level with white chocolate and bits of dried fruit.*

1. Melt the butter and chocolate together in a double boiler over just-simmering water. When melted, remove from the heat and set aside to cool.

2. Preheat the oven to 350°F. Lightly butter an 8-inch or 9-inch cake pan.

3. Beat together the sugar and egg until light and fluffy. Beat in the vanilla. Combine the flour, baking powder, and salt in a separate bowl and beat with the sugar mixture until just incorporated. Stir in the butter-chocolate mixture gently and the 2 different berries until just incorporated. Spoon the batter into the prepared pan.

4. Bake the blondies for about 25 minutes or until the center feels firm and a toothpick inserted in the center comes out clean. Cool on a rack before slicing.

Sautéed Bananas, Jackfruit, and Toddy Palm with Rum-Coconut Cream

A simple yet showy dessert, this lush tropical mixture can grace even a formal meal. Look for the toddy palm and jackfruit combo in cans at an Asian market.

1. Heat the butter in a large skillet over medium heat and when it is melted and bubbly, stir in the brown sugar, mixing well. When that is hot and bubbly, stir in the coconut milk to combine.

2. Stir in the bananas and the jackfruit-toddy palm mixture and cook, stirring, for about 4 minutes. Stir in the rum, mixing well. Serve hot.

What Are Toddy Palm and Jackfruit?

From the tropical toddy palm tree—the sap from this palm variety is used to make the potent brew—the toddy palm (as you find it named in the marketplace) is the immature and translucent seeds; they have a pleasingly soft gelatinous texture and gentle sweetness that is alluring. The jackfruit, also from the tropics, is a large, spiny-skinned fruit with an orange flesh that tastes like a cross between a mango and a banana. The fruit may be sold fresh, but it's tricky to open and extract the fruit. It's readily available canned at most Asian markets.

SERVES 4

410 calories
15g fat
67g carbohydrates
2g protein
25mg sodium
5g fiber

INGREDIENTS:
3 tablespoons butter
3 tablespoons brown sugar
½ cup coconut milk
3 bananas, peeled and sliced on the diagonal
1 (20-ounce) can mixed sliced jackfruit and whole toddy palm in liquid, well drained
3 tablespoons rum, or more as desired

420 calories
16g fat
67g carbohydrates
4g protein
105mg sodium
3g fiber

INGREDIENTS:

*3 cups chopped fresh or frozen
  rhubarb*
*2 cups canned crushed
  pineapple, well drained*
1 cup sugar
2 tablespoons cornstarch
*1 sheet frozen puff pastry,
  thawed*

Margo's Rhubarb and Pineapple Tart

*This unusual dessert is just fine if served plain, but adding
whipped cream or vanilla ice cream elevates it to another
dimension.*

1. Preheat the oven to 350°F.

2. Combine the rhubarb, pineapple, sugar, and cornstarch in a large
   mixing bowl, mixing well. On a lightly floured surface, roll out the
   sheet of puff pastry just enough to fit into a deep 1½-quart baking
   dish. Press it into the dish and fill it with the fruit mixture. Fold the
   corners in toward the center.

3. Bake the tart for about 40 minutes or until the crust has puffed and
   turned brown. Serve it hot or still warm.

Watermelon Dessert Soup

To achieve maximum effect, be sure to use only a very ripe, sweet watermelon. If the seductive lemon flavor of the liqueur appeals, add more to taste.

1. Cut up the watermelon half into cubes and put them into a blender. Add the pomegranate juice and limoncello and process until smooth. Chill.

2. Pour 1 cup per serving into 4 individual soup bowls. Swirl 1 table-spoon heavy cream into each serving. Add ½ cup melon balls per serving and top with mint leaves as desired.

What Is Limoncello?

An Italian lemon liqueur, limoncello has a delightfully spirited citrus taste, delicious on its own or added as a flavor enhancer to sweets. In Italy, it's often served as an after-dinner digestive. For its fans, limoncello is apparently easy to make at home—with the right ingredients.

SERVE 4

370 calories
6g fat
86g carbohydrates
3g protein
40mg sodium
5g fiber

INGREDIENTS:

*½ small seedless watermelon
   plus extra for melon balls
½ cup pomegranate juice
¼ cup limoncello
¼ cup heavy cream
2 cups melon balls for garnish
Mint leaves for garnish*

CHAPTER 15

Sweet Endings

Whether you are a vegetarian or not, desserts have universal appeal. Even people counting calories or sugar grams can put a cheerful exclamation point at the end of the meal by enjoying luscious ripened and seasonal fruits drizzled with lime juice or a splash of pomegranate juice. In other words, desserts may often be calorie traps, but they don't have to end up that way.

15

Healthful Desserts

Can desserts be good for you? Healthful? Are desserts and health a contradiction in terms? That all depends on what and how much you eat. Of course, eating in moderation means you can have your cake, pudding, and even pie and enjoy every mouthful when the occasion merits it. The savvy consumer knows when indulgences are allowable, how to downsize portions, and when to skip that extra fatty calorie for something fruity and delicate.

And in this age of going green, the wise cook looks for the dessert basics among the good-for-you ingredients, such as unrefined flours and sugars, butter instead of hydrogenated fats, organically grown fruits, and primo flavorings and spices.

Counting Calories . . . and Making Calories Count

Of course, calories do count and add up fast. Anyone who keeps up with health news must know that America is becoming a nation of the obese, a fact that the CDC confirms: about 34 percent of American adults are overweight or obese, and the figures for overweight youngsters are climbing steadily.

As the CDC reports, overweight and obesity are major causes of chronic health problems, including type 2 diabetes, high blood pressure, coronary heart disease and stroke, and osteoarthritis. Fortunately for those on the basically low-fat and high-fiber vegetarian eating plan, overweight and its consequences can be diminished if not totally avoided.

Add calorie counting and food wisdom to a vibrant exercise plan and you end up with a decent shot at good health. And if you are really concerned about weight gain, check with your doctor to determine what your ideal weight is, based on age, sex, general health, and activity level—then map out your menus and eat accordingly, adding a dessert for just the right occasion. To see a suggested calorie-balanced meal plan for lacto-ovó vegetarians, go to *www.nhlbi.nih.gov/health/public/heart/obesity/lose_wt/lacto_ov.htm*.

Sugars and Natural and Artificial Sweeteners

Americans seem to have the world's largest sweet tooth, and according to the USDA, we have the largest sweetener market in the world, consuming quantities of high fructose corn syrup and sugars processed from sugar beets and sugarcane.

What Are Sugars?

Sugar occurs naturally in starches as the end product of metabolism. Common forms of sugars are glucose, or blood sugar; sucrose, the sugars used in cooking; dextrose, or corn sugar; fructose; lactose or milk sugar, and maltose, or malt sugar. Because sugar is a carbohydrate, it is also a source of energy needed to fuel every organ and to keep muscles working smoothly. Table sugar, or sucrose, is made up of a bonding between glucose and fructose.

But naturally occurring sugars are one thing; added sugars are something else entirely. The numerous forms of sugars added to such foods as baked goods, soda pops, and many processed foods are posing health problems—particularly obesity and its concurrent risk of type 2 diabetes and tooth decay—because they can boost sugar intake to excessive levels.

According to the Institute of Medicine's Dietary Reference Intakes (DRI) Report, Americans should get the majority of their daily calories from carbohydrates—about 45 to 65 percent of their daily calories. The DRI for carbohydrates and sugars recommends a maximum intake level of 25 percent or less from added sugars.

Figuring out what is an added sugar makes reading labels important: you'll know sugar has been added when you see listed such ingredients as high fructose corn syrup, corn syrup, dextrose, fructose, fruit juice concentrates, honey, and malt syrup. As in everything else, moderation is key.

Other Natural Sweeteners

Vegans generally avoid using refined sugars because some sugars from sugar cane may have been processed with animal bone char; however, modern technology has advanced so far that most sugars are whitened by other means, and refined sugar made from sugar beets or natural raw sugar has never been processed with bone char. (Note that vegans also do not use honey.) If you are looking for a sweetener other than refined sugar, you have plenty of options, including agave syrup, maple syrup, date sugar, evaporated cane juice, fructose, brown rice syrup, molasses, stevia, and raw sugar.

Sugar Substitutes

Whether they are friend or foe, artificial sweeteners, also known as sugar substitutes, are chemicals that form a product that sweetens without adding discernable calories. For diabetics and dieters, these products are a real boon. But not every food labeled "sugar free" is calorie free, or even totally sugar free. The sweetener sorbitol, for example, contains calories, so it can have an effect on your blood sugar.

The FDA has approved four sugar substitutes, or sweeteners, that are safe—and sweet—and currently on the market. These include saccharin, aspartame, sucralose (sold as the product Splenda), and acesulfame potassium. If taken in moderate amounts, none pose health risks, not even saccharin, once thought to be linked to certain cancers.

Flour Power

If you are a baker or simply a home cook who uses flour for thickening gravies or coating foods for frying, you know that flour in all its many guises is a kitchen staple. You probably pick up a bag of flour fairly regularly, but with so many choices on the market, what should you look for?

Types of Flour

Perhaps the best news for bakers who want a quality baked good with a delicate texture is the arrival of unbleached white whole wheat flours on market shelves. Ground from white whole wheat, these flours have all the nutritional benefits of the standard whole wheat flours but without their earthy flavor and the crumbly texture they impart to baked goods. Using white whole wheat flour, gradually at first if you wish, helps boost the health value of home-baked goods, from waffles to muffins.

Unless you bake breads or cakes and need specific bread or cake flours, you should choose an all-purpose flour, preferably unbleached and enriched—and from organic wheat—for most baking methods. Whole wheat flour milled from red wheat berries with the bran and germ intact provides needed nutrients, but the flour tends to turn rancid fast.

Other useful—and nutritious—flours include rye flour, oat flour, and soy flour. Note that soy flour is not used as the main flour in a recipe; it is only added as a way to supplement the protein content of baked goods, such as bread, and to provide a nutty taste and darker color.

Fats and Oils

Most folks cringe at the word *fat*, yet everyone needs some dietary fat for good health and energy. The fats and oils used in cooking and at the table, however, should be selected wisely and used sparingly.

Butters and Margarines

If you check out the Internet, you'll find that the "butter versus margarine" controversies have been long and passionate. In a nutshell, it's all about saturated fats (butter) as opposed to trans fats and some saturated fats (margarines). And depending on whose information you read, one is definitely better or worse for you than the other. In the end, eating a natural product, butter, despite its saturated fats, is probably a safer choice than most margarines with their trans fats. Note that some brands of margarine, including soy-based margarines and "buttery" spreads, are free of trans fats and partially hydrogenated oils.

So when you read the label and see that a product contains "hydrogenated fat"—which has hydrogen molecules added to the fat to increase its meltability and prevent its turning rancid—you should read that as "trans fats." These fats have been linked to heart disease by raising the levels of bad cholesterol in your blood.

The Oils

Which are the good fats, the ones that improve cholesterol levels in the blood, the ones that are plant based in origin? If you've followed the fat controversy, you'll know you'll want to stock up on the unsaturated-fat oils such as olive oil, canola oil, and peanut oils.

You'll also know that unsaturated fats are divided into two categories: monounsaturated fats from olive oil, nuts, seeds and avocados; and polyunsaturated fats, from sunflower, corn, soybean, and flaxseed oils. Oils in either category are better for you than saturated fats. Nevertheless, the USDA recommends using fats and oils sparingly and substituting fat-free or low-fat dressings for salads. And remember, all fats, regardless of the source, contain the same number of calories gram per gram.

Good olive oils—that is, extra virgin oils from the first pressing of the olive—are particularly valued in the kitchen for their full, fruity flavors that impart a seductive accent and fragrance to dressings and garnishes. Less expensive virgin olive oils are fine for sautéing and cooking, but no olive oil really stands up well to the high-heat requirements of stir-frying or deep-frying.

Besides its distinctive flavor and its lack of saturated fat, olive oil has long been favored for its possible assorted medicinal and health properties, from supporting longevity among those on a Mediterranean oil-and-vegetable-and-salad diet to being a heart-healthy food to lowering blood pressure to banishing wrinkles.

Chocolate and Other Flavorings

Almost every dish you cook can benefit by a careful addition of flavors, seasonings, spices, herbs, and extracts.

Chocolate, the Feel-Good Flavor

When it comes down to cooking a dish calling for that best flavoring of all, chocolate, you can indulge your sweet tooth without too many qualms. For the good news is: chocolates, especially the darker ones, may actually help lower blood pressure and may, with their antioxidants, boost your immune system.

That's added reasons to celebrate, for chocolate lovers are a passionate group, and are happy to find any good excuse to add this ingredient to their daily diet. The problem is that most chocolates are processed with fat from cocoa butter and sugar to sweeten the bitter cacao powder. What's a chocoholic to do? Eat moderately.

The best chocolate for baking or cooking needs will depend on what you plan to make. There are many domestic and imported chocolates and cocoas available. Whichever you select, store your chocolate in a cool, dry place away from heat and your product should last for a long time. To learn more about this best-loved ingredient, check out *www.chocolateusa.org*.

Extracts and Spices

In desserts, pure extracts and freshly ground spices add an element of flavor that completes the picture. Liquid extracts and spices do deteriorate after opening, and you should discard any opened liquids after one year.

Whole spices, if frozen, may retain their flavors for at least one year. Ground spices may retain their spark for up to six months, but before you use them, do the sniff-and-look test: if there is no fragrance, or they have lost their vibrant color, discard them. Don't try to use outdated spices, as they may impart an unpleasant taste. If possible, grind whole spices just before use. Store ground spices in a cool, dry place.

680 calories
32g fat
86g carbohydrates
12g protein
270mg sodium
1g fiber

INGREDIENTS:

*1 (14-ounce) can coconut milk,
    well chilled*

*1 (14-ounce) can sweetened
    condensed milk*

*1 (16.8-ounce) bottle passion
    fruit concentrate*

2 cups cubed pound cake

1 cup toasted shredded coconut

*Fresh fruits such as cut-up
    strawberries or blueberries
    as garnish*

Brazilian-Style Passion Fruit Pudding

*For best results, chill the coconut milk before use, and then use
only the thickened top cream—do not include the thin coconut
water at the bottom of the can. The acidic quality of the fruit
thickens the mixture until it becomes firm.*

1. Carefully scoop out the thick layer of coconut milk and put it into a
    bowl. Beat the milk until it thickens and resembles partially whipped
    heavy cream. Stir in the condensed milk. Fill the condensed milk
    can with the passion fruit concentrate and pour it into the mixing
    bowl. Stir well to combine the milks and juice.

2. Line the bottom of a 2-quart dessert bowl with the pound cake.
    Pour the passion fruit mixture over top and chill until firm. To serve,
    sprinkle the toasted coconut over the mousse, spoon the mixture
    into individual bowls, and garnish with fresh fruits as desired.

What Is Passion Fruit?

A tropical fruit native to Brazil, passion fruit has a subtle sweetness and
perfume that only enhances its appeal. Its nectar is often blended into a
fruit drink and a passion fruit concentrate, which you need for this recipe,
is readily available at Hispanic markets. You may also find a frozen concentrate, but it does not produce the same results.

Chocolate Tofu Pudding

This very easy-to-make pudding tastes like an extravagantly decadent mousse with loads of cream, but its rich texture— and extra protein—come from tofu. If you want to reduce calories, omit the chocolate chips, making this dessert an even healthier choice. Be sure to use the "cook-and-serve" puddings, not the instant ones.

1. Combine the milk, tofu, and pudding mixture in a blender and process until smooth. Pour the mixture into a saucepane. Heat slowly over medium-low heat, stirring constantly, until the mixture thickens.

2. Remove from the heat, stir in the chocolate bits, and pour into a heatproof bowl. Chill until ready to serve.

SERVES 4

340 calories
14g fat
51g carbohydrates
10g protein
150mg sodium
3g fiber

INGREDIENTS:

2 cups nonfat milk or soymilk
1½ cups silken firm tofu
2 (1.3-ounce) boxes sugar-free and fat-free chocolate pudding mixture
1 cup chocolate chips

SERVES 8

910 calories
58g fat
88g carbohydrates
15g protein
490mg sodium
2g fiber

INGREDIENTS:

2 cups crushed gingersnaps
4 tablespoons butter, melted
2 tablespoons freshly grated
    fresh ginger
2 tablespoons brown sugar
2 pounds cream cheese, at room
    temperature
2 cups granulated sugar, or to
    taste
4 large eggs
2 tablespoons cornstarch
2 teaspoons vanilla extract
Pinch salt
½ cup shredded coconut
½ cup diced dried papaya
½ cup thinly sliced almonds

Tropical Cheesecake

Here's another dessert that lends itself to variations: instead of diced papaya, you may substitute diced dried pineapple or mango and use crushed macadamia nuts instead of almonds. And to cut calories, try using a reduced-fat cream cheese.

1. Preheat the oven to 325°F. Combine the crushed gingersnaps and the butter and press the mixture into the bottom of a 10-inch springform pan. Sprinkle the grated ginger and brown sugar on top of the crumbs, pressing them into the crust.

2. Beat the cream cheese and sugar until smooth. Beat in eggs one at a time until well combined and add cornstarch, vanilla extract, and salt. Stir in the fruit by hand.

3. Pour half the mixture onto the crust, sprinkle a layer of almonds on top, and pour on the remaining mixture.

4. Bake for at least 1 hour and 20 minutes or until the center is firm; turn off the heat but leave the cheesecake in the oven until it is cool. Then refrigerate it for at least 12 hours before slicing.

Berry-Streusel Tart

This dessert is so easy to make that you may use it often, especially when last-minute friends drop by and want something sweet at the end of the meal. The crust and streusel are based on prepackaged sugar cookie dough, which adds to its speedy preparation. You can serve this hot or cold and add ice cream or a whipped topping, as you wish.

1. Preheat the oven to 350°F. Lightly butter and flour an 8" × 8" or 9" × 9" round or square cake pan.

2. Slice the cookie dough into two portions, using ¾ of the dough for the crust. Press the dough into the bottom of the pan. Combine the flour and the remaining cookie dough, crumbling the mixture with your fingertips; set aside. In a separate bowl, toss the berries with the granulated sugar, cornstarch, and almond extract, if using, and spoon the mixture into the pan. Sprinkle the streusel mixture evenly over top.

3. Bake for about 40 minutes or until the top has turned brown and the center feels firm. Remove from the oven and eat hot or cold.

SERVES 6

450 calories
17g fat
71g carbohydrates
5g protein
330mg sodium
3g fiber

INGREDIENTS:
1 (16½-ounce) package sugar
  cookie dough
½ cup all-purpose flour
3 cups fresh or frozen mixed
  berries
¼ cup granulated sugar
2 tablespoons cornstarch
1 teaspoon almond extract,
  optional

**MAKES ABOUT 16
(3-INCH) CUPCAKES**

290 calories
20g fat
27g carbohydrates
4g protein
75mg sodium
2g fiber

INGREDIENTS:

4 ounces unsweetened
   chocolate squares
½ pound (2 sticks) unsalted
   butter
6 large eggs
1 cup granulated sugar
¾ cup cake flour
1½ teaspoons baking powder
2 teaspoons vanilla extract
1 tablespoon cocoa powder
Pinch salt
1 cup mini chocolate morsels

Triple-Chocolate Cupcakes

*A cross between a brownie and a muffin, these elegant
chocolate morsels have an intense chocolate flavor heightened
by the cocoa powder.*

1. Preheat the oven to 350°F. Spray nonstick muffin cups with nonstick cooking spray. Melt the chocolate and butter together over low heat. When melted, cool to room temperature.

2. Meanwhile, beat the eggs with the sugar until the mixture turns a pale lemon-yellow. Spoon the cooled chocolate mixture into the sugar-egg mixture and stir until combined. Stir in the cake flour, baking powder, vanilla extract, cocoa powder, and salt and beat for about 30 seconds. Stir in the chocolate morsels. Spoon the mixture into the cups until each is about two-thirds full.

3. Bake 15 to 18 minutes or until a toothpick inserted in the center comes out clean and the cupcakes feel firm. Cool completely.

Ginger-Tapioca Pudding

A lively ginger syrup adds a hint of the exotic to this old-fashioned favorite. To make the syrup, use about 2 inches fresh ginger thinly sliced and cooked with ½ cup brown sugar in 1 cup water. Boil this mixture for about 5 minutes, cool, and strain, discarding the ginger.

1. Combine the tapioca, ginger syrup, and coconut milk and pour into a large saucepan. Beat stir in the eggs and heat over medium-low heat, stirring constantly as the mixture begins to thicken.

2. Meanwhile, sprinkle the crumbled macaroons into the bottom of a 1½-quart dessert dish.

3. When the tapioca pudding has thickened, spoon it into the dessert dish and completely chill until firm.

What Is Pearl Tapioca?

The old-fashioned tapioca pudding called for using the regular, not instant, pearl tapioca made from the starch of the cassava plant. Larger and harder than the instant tapioca pearls, these require soaking for at least 12 hours, but preferably for up to 24 hours. Otherwise, they never quite soften during cooking. Despite this advance planning, the pudding is really worth the effort.

SERVES 4

520 calories
25g fat
73g carbohydrates
6g protein
150mg sodium
2g fiber

INGREDIENTS:
½ cup pearl tapioca soaked in
    1 cup water for at least 12
    hours
1 cup ginger syrup
1½ cups coconut milk
2 eggs, well beaten
Pinch salt
6 coconut macaroons, crumbled

SERVES 4

360 calories
0g fat
95g carbohydrates
1g protein
60mg sodium
3g fiber

INGREDIENTS:

Juice of 3 limes
1 tablespoon freshly grated
fresh ginger
3 ripe mangoes, peeled and
sliced
1 teaspoon fresh lime zest
1 cup sugar syrup (see sidebar)

Mango-Ginger Ice

Select ripe mangoes, preferably the flat yellow varieties
available seasonally. These have a subtle sweet flavor that
works well with fresh ginger.

Combine the ingredients in the container of a blender and process
until smooth. Chill the mixture and churn according to manufacturer's directions. Scoop the mixture into a container and freeze.

How Do I Make a Simple Sugar Syrup?

To make sugar syrup: Combine 3 cups water and 2 cups granulated sugar
in a saucepan and cook over medium-low heat until the sugar dissolves
entirely and the mixture turns slightly syrupy. Set aside to cool. Save leftovers for another use.

Ultra Chocolate-Mint Tart

For a totally different take on the filling, use a soy cream cheese instead of the regular one. Whichever you use, this tastes like a ritzy cheesecake.

1. Preheat the oven to 350°F.

2. Combine the vegetable oil and the chocolate squares in the top of a double boiler and melt the chocolate over just-simmering water. Set aside to cool slightly.

3. Meanwhile, beat together the cream cheese, sugar, and cornstarch until smooth. Beat in the eggs one at a time. Stir in the cocoa, brandy, and melted chocolate. Spoon the mixture into the shell. Sprinkle the top with the mint-chocolate bits.

4. Bake the tart for about 1 hour or until the center is firm. Remove from the oven and cool. Before serving, sprinkle with confectioners' sugar.

SERVES 6

670 calories
51g fat
49g carbohydrates
13g protein
370mg sodium
5g fiber

INGREDIENTS:

1 tablespoon vegetable oil
4 ounces semisweet chocolate squares
1 pound cream cheese, at room temperature
½ cup unsifted confectioners' sugar
2 tablespoons cornstarch
2 large eggs
1 tablespoon unsweetened cocoa
1 tablespoon brandy
1 9-inch ready-made chocolate cookie crumb crust
½ cup mint-chocolate bits
Confectioners' sugar for sprinkling

SERVES 4

710 calories
49g fat
74g carbohydrates
6g protein
90mg sodium
6g fiber

INGREDIENTS:
½ cup small sago pearls or pearl
    tapioca
2 fresh or frozen pandan leaves,
    knotted together
4 cups coconut milk
2 to 3 yellow-ripe plantains,
    peeled and cut on the
    diagonal into 2-inch lengths
2 to 2½ tablespoons sugar, or
    to taste
¼ teaspoon salt
Crushed peanuts for garnish

Brigitte's Vietnamese Tapioca Pudding

*If you cannot find sago pearls, which soften in boiled water in
about 5 minutes, you'll need to soak the larger pearl tapioca
overnight before use. You can serve this pudding warm, room
temperature, or cold, and this makes a delicious breakfast
treat.*

1. Bring 2 cups water to a boil, remove from the heat, and soak the ½
    cup sago pearls.

2. Meanwhile, heat the pandan leaves in the coconut milk and bring
    to a boil over medium heat. Add the sago or tapioca and reduce the
    heat to low. Add the plantains and stir in the sugar and salt. Continue
    cooking for about 5 minutes. Remove from the heat, discard the
    pandan leaves, and serve or set aside for later use. Before serving,
    sprinkle the pudding with crushed peanuts.

What Is Pandan?
Pandan leaves, beloved by many Southeast Asians for the distinctive pale
green it lends to the cooked dish and for its unforgettable, delicate piney
aroma and flavor, are sold frozen and sometimes fresh in Asian markets.
In many Asian markets, you can even find pandan extract, known as
kewra, and if all else fails, simply substitute vanilla extract. Because the
leaves are long, cooks typically knot them together before adding them
to the cookpot.

Cantaloupe-Peach Soup

Best when melons and peaches are at their prime, this refreshing soup is both light and delicate, an ideal summer dessert. Slices of angel food cake add the final finishing touch.

1. Combine the cantaloupe, peaches, guava nectar, lime juice, and sugar in a blender or food processor and purée until smooth. Chill.

2. To serve, spoon the soup into individual bowls and garnish with strawberry slices.

SERVES 4

140 calories
0g fat
36g carbohydrates
2g protein
15mg sodium
3g fiber

INGREDIENTS:
2 cups cubed cantaloupe
2 cups cubed peaches
1½ cups guava nectar
2 tablespoons fresh lime juice
2 tablespoons sugar, or to taste
Sliced strawberries for garnish

APPENDIX

Resources

Resources for New Vegetarians

Perhaps the most complete American website is that of the Vegetarian Resource Group. The group provides an answer for almost any question a vegetarian can think of. The staff is also willing to help out by phone or e-mail.

www.vrg.org

Resources for Concerned Parents

Vegetarian parents have plenty of resources to help them create healthful lifestyles for their family. For general dietary guidelines, you should study the USDA's dietary guidelines and review the Nemours Foundation's recommendations; see below.

Also visit:

www.kidshealth.org

www.vegfamily.com

You can also turn to the website of the American Academy of Pediatrics, including such links as:

http://aappolicy.aappublications.org/cgi/content/full/pediatrics;115/2/496

www.aap.org/publiced/BR_Solids.htm

http://aappolicy.aappublications.org/cgi/content/full/pediatrics;117/2/544

Resources for Going Green, Thinking Green

Many websites address the most common issues that concerned consumers may have about environmental issues and working for safer food sources. The following are good places to start:

www.localharvest.org

www.slowfoodusa.org

The Sierra Club

www.sierraclub.org

The Nature Conservancy

www.nature.org

The Orion Grassroots Network

www.orionsociety.org

American Farmland Trust

www.farmland.org

Resources for Parents of Young Children

Many vegetarian and vegan parents are already acquainted with food plans and the nutritional needs of their youngsters, but besides consulting their child's pediatrician, reading up on how best to feed children for their maximum health is a wise decision for all parents. A good place to start is at this website:

http://kidshealth.org/parent/nutrition_fit/nutrition/vegetarianism.html

Other sources of sound information include:

The Vegetarian Resource Group

www.vrg.org

The USDA's website, where parents can see what comprises a sound diet

www.mypyramid.gov

The Vegetarian Society's website, which details nutritional information geared to specific age groups.

www.vegsoc.org/info/childre1.html

Resources for Teens

Tapping into the growing trend of teens getting interested in vegetarianism and turning to a meat-free diet, several authorities have put together information to help teens follow a healthful vegetarian lifestyle. The following sites offer valuable information and tips specifically aimed at teens.

www.vegetarianteen.com

Vegetarian Resource Group's website:

www.vrg.org/nutrition/teennutrition.htm

Compiled by the Nemours Foundation

http://kidshealth.org/teen/food_fitness/nutrition/vegetarian.html

Resources for General Interest Consumers

Perhaps the most comprehensive collection of information is available from the National Agricultural Library USDA, published in April 2008. Entitled *Vegetarian Nutrition Resource List*, this twenty-five-page document provides names of articles, pamphlets, and books covering vegetarian nutrition, plus suggestions on ways to obtain the various materials. The list is available from the Food and Nutrition Information Center's website at:

www.nal.usda.gov/fnic/resource_lists.shtml

Resources for Vegetarian Food Products

Many major supermarkets and health food markets now stock a wide range of all-veg products, from "cheeses" and "yogurts" to "sausages" and "ground meat" look-alikes. But consumers can also track down a warehouse full of items most markets may not stock—then request management stock them or order them online. Other options for locating vegetarian food products is to go to the website of your favorite food manufacturer, and order directly from them. For sources of shippable food items, the Internet is a treasure trove.

Vegetarians in Paradise

www.vegparadise.com/foodmakers.html

Fantastic Foods

An all-natural, all-vegetarian food manufacturer of such product as soups, entrées, international dishes, and couscous and rice.

www.fantasticfoods.com

Vegefood

This website purports to have the lartest online selection of vegetarian food, so chances are that you'll find everything you want in one location. Go to:

www.vegefood.com

The Vegan Store

Selling Pangea vegan foods and a host of all-vegan and cruelty-free housewares, clothing, and office products, plus much more, this site has a question-answer section for people asking about all-vegan goods. The Pangea staff is located in Rockville, Maryland, but consumers can order all their products online at:

www.veganstore.com

EcoBusinessLinks

For vegetarians/vegans who want "green" and organic goods, this website tells consumers not only which stores are located in which states, but also lists organic farms and organic food suppliers, not all of which are vegetarian. Visit:

www.ecobusinesslinks.com

Melissa's

Having made its fame and fortune by providing consumers with top-quality, and often unusual, produce, Melissa's also offer a line of soy-based vegetarian ingredients, including ready-to-eat organic edamame, organic soy nuts, soy slices, soy tacos, and an exhilarating soy chorizo, a Mexican-inspired spicy sausage mixture. To find store locations or to order online visit:

www.melissas.com

Additional Resources

American Dietetic Association

With more than 68,000 members as of this writing, the American Dietetic Association (ADA) is the world's largest group of dietary professionals. Its members are involved in all aspects of the field of nutrition and health, including research and education. Its booklet *Becoming Vegetarian* (2007) outlines the fundamentals of a basic vegetarian diet and provides tips on how to eat out vegetarian and ways to shift to a vegetarian way of eating.

www.eatright.org

International Vegetarian Union (IVU)

The acknowledged grandfather of the international vegetarian movement, the IVU came into being in the early 1900s in Germany during the first vegetarian congress. A nonprofit group, its sole purpose is to promote vegetarianism worldwide, a goal they want to achieve by holding regular congresses, answering questions, dispensing diets and recipes, and maintaining an archive on vegetarian-based information.

www.ivu.org

Moosewood Restaurant

Upstate New York restaurant under the aegis of Moosewood Inc., which is commonly credited with kicking off the boom of vegetarianism in the United States. The restaurant, which opened in Ithaca in the early 1970s, certainly took vegetarian cooking and ideals and made them palatable and interesting to a new generation of Americans. As a collective, the restaurant's staff wrote and published the original *Moosewood Cookbook*, which attracted both fame and notoriety to the place.

www.moosewoodrestaurant.com

Oldways Preservation Trust

Founded in the 1980s by Bostonian K. Dun Gifford, the Oldways organization has as its mission simplifying nutritional science and converting food facts into palate-pleasing fare. Gifford and colleague Sara Baer-Sinnott have initiated numerous food-related activities and conferences to promote better health through better diets. Its staff have also developed consumer materials, including several diet pyramids and a cookbook entitled *The Oldways Table*.

www.oldwayspt.org

The Vegetarian Society of the United Kingdom

Formed in England in 1847, the society is the longest-running all-vegetarian group in the world, espousing and supporting an all-vegetarian lifestyle that includes many levels of activities, from fund-raising, lecturing, and providing nutritional advice to creating recipes and teaching cooking. The group also established and runs the annual National Vegetarian Week with concurrent activities.

www.vegsoc.org

Vegetarian Resource Group (VRG)

The VRG is a source of vegetarian information, vegetarian (actually, vegan) recipes, and a resource for all aspects of a vegetarian lifestyle, with even a listing of vegetarian travel services and tips on how to order vegetarian when dining out. In addition to its very complete website, the VRG has archived numerous vegetarian-based articles and has published vegan cookbooks as well as a newsletter and a magazine entitled *The Vegetarian Journal*.

www.vrg.org

Natural Food Supplies

Nature's Harvest
P.O. 291, 28 Main Street, Blairstown, NJ 07825
Contact Michelle St. Andre: 908-362-6766
Harvest6766@embarqmail.com

Organic Produce
www.diamondorganics.com

Whole Grains and Sea Vegetables
www.kushistore.com/acatalog/welcome.html

Organic foods and products
www.diamondorganics.com

Vegetables, Earthbound Farm
www.ebfarm.com

Cascadian Farms, frozen fruits and vegetables
www.cfarm.com

Seeds of Change, organic tomato sauces and salsas
www.seedsofchange.com

Green Mountain Coffee Roasters
(organic, sustainably grown, fair trade)
www.greenmountaincoffee.com

Health Education Websites

Dr. Joseph Mercola
www.mercola.com

Organic Consumers Association
www.organicconsumers.org

Energy Consumption Statistics

Energy Information Administration Website
www.eia.doe.gov/kids/classactivities/CrunchTheNumbersIntermediat-eDec2002.pdf

USGS Website
http://energy.cr.usgs.gov/energy/stats_ctry/Stat1.htmla

U.S. Department of Energy's division of energy efficiency and renewable energy
www.eere.gov

Saving with Recycling, NRDC Website
www.nrdc.org/land/forests/gtissue.asp

Saving with Compact Fluorescents, Environmental Defense Website
www.environmentaldefense.org/article.cfm?contentid=5215

Sustainable Building and Retrofitting

Bob Swain's Website
www.bobswain.com

General building information
www.greenbuilder.com

Alternative energy systems, products, and installation
www.utilityfree.com

Saline Pool Systems
www.salinepoolsystems.com

Sick Building Syndrome
www.wellbuilding.com

Renewable Resources

www.green-e.org

www.greenfacts.org

www.greentagusa.org

Other Resources

Cleaning Chemicals
www.restoreproducts.com

Tom Foerstel's Website for organic products
www.organic.org
www.organiclinks.com

Daliya Robson's Website for nontoxic household furnishings
www.nontoxic.com

For sustainably harvested household products
www.seventhgeneration.com

Teflon
www.tuberose.com/Teflon.html

Chemical-free home products
www.EnvironProducts.com

Measuring your environmental footprint
www.carbonfootprint.com

What the labels really say
truthinlabeling.org

Index

Note: Page numbers in *italics* indicate recipes.

W

Waffles, *61*
Woks, 42
World Vegan Day, 10
World Vegetarian Day, 10
Wraps, *84*

Y

Yogurt. *See also* Smoothies
about: benefits of, 58; making
yogurt cheese, 58
Banana-Pineapple-Yogurt Frosty,
237
Fried Chickpeas with Yogurt, *126*

Z

Zinc, 14, 23, 55, 73, 75–76

THE EVERYTHING SERIES!

BUSINESS & PERSONAL FINANCE

Everything® Accounting Book
Everything® Budgeting Book, 2nd Ed.
Everything® Business Planning Book
Everything® Coaching and Mentoring Book, 2nd Ed.
Everything® Fundraising Book
Everything® Get Out of Debt Book
Everything® Grant Writing Book, 2nd Ed.
Everything® Guide to Buying Foreclosures
Everything® Guide to Fundraising, $15.95
Everything® Guide to Mortgages
Everything® Guide to Personal Finance for Single Mothers
Everything® Home-Based Business Book, 2nd Ed.
Everything® Homebuying Book, 3rd Ed., $15.95
Everything® Homeselling Book, 2nd Ed.
Everything® Human Resource Management Book
Everything® Improve Your Credit Book
Everything® Investing Book, 2nd Ed.
Everything® Landlording Book
Everything® Leadership Book, 2nd Ed.
Everything® Managing People Book, 2nd Ed.
Everything® Negotiating Book
Everything® Online Auctions Book
Everything® Online Business Book
Everything® Personal Finance Book
Everything® Personal Finance in Your 20s & 30s Book, 2nd Ed.
Everything® Personal Finance in Your 40s & 50s Book, $15.95
Everything® Project Management Book, 2nd Ed.
Everything® Real Estate Investing Book
Everything® Retirement Planning Book
Everything® Robert's Rules Book, $7.95
Everything® Selling Book
Everything® Start Your Own Business Book, 2nd Ed.
Everything® Wills & Estate Planning Book

COOKING

Everything® Barbecue Cookbook
Everything® Bartender's Book, 2nd Ed., $9.95
Everything® Calorie Counting Cookbook
Everything® Cheese Book
Everything® Chinese Cookbook
Everything® Classic Recipes Book
Everything® Cocktail Parties & Drinks Book
Everything® College Cookbook
Everything® Cooking for Baby and Toddler Book
Everything® Diabetes Cookbook
Everything® Easy Gourmet Cookbook
Everything® Fondue Cookbook
Everything® Food Allergy Cookbook, $15.95
Everything® Fondue Party Book
Everything® Gluten-Free Cookbook
Everything® Glycemic Index Cookbook
Everything® Grilling Cookbook
Everything® Healthy Cooking for Parties Book, $15.95
Everything® Holiday Cookbook
Everything® Indian Cookbook
Everything® Lactose-Free Cookbook
Everything® Low-Cholesterol Cookbook

Everything® Low-Fat High-Flavor Cookbook, 2nd Ed., $15.95
Everything® Low-Salt Cookbook
Everything® Meals for a Month Cookbook
Everything® Meals on a Budget Cookbook
Everything® Mediterranean Cookbook
Everything® Mexican Cookbook
Everything® No Trans Fat Cookbook
Everything® One-Pot Cookbook, 2nd Ed., $15.95
Everything® Organic Cooking for Baby & Toddler Book, $15.95
Everything® Pizza Cookbook
Everything® Quick Meals Cookbook, 2nd Ed., $15.95
Everything® Slow Cooker Cookbook
Everything® Slow Cooking for a Crowd Cookbook
Everything® Soup Cookbook
Everything® Stir-Fry Cookbook
Everything® Sugar-Free Cookbook
Everything® Tapas and Small Plates Cookbook
Everything® Tex-Mex Cookbook
Everything® Thai Cookbook
Everything® Vegetarian Cookbook
Everything® Whole-Grain, High-Fiber Cookbook
Everything® Wild Game Cookbook
Everything® Wine Book, 2nd Ed.

GAMES

Everything® 15-Minute Sudoku Book, $9.95
Everything® 30-Minute Sudoku Book, $9.95
Everything® Bible Crosswords Book, $9.95
Everything® Blackjack Strategy Book
Everything® Brain Strain Book, $9.95
Everything® Bridge Book
Everything® Card Games Book
Everything® Card Tricks Book, $9.95
Everything® Casino Gambling Book, 2nd Ed.
Everything® Chess Basics Book
Everything® Christmas Crosswords Book, $9.95
Everything® Craps Strategy Book
Everything® Crossword and Puzzle Book
Everything® Crosswords and Puzzles for Quote Lovers Book, $9.95
Everything® Crossword Challenge Book
Everything® Crosswords for the Beach Book, $9.95
Everything® Cryptic Crosswords Book, $9.95
Everything® Cryptograms Book, $9.95
Everything® Easy Crosswords Book
Everything® Easy Kakuro Book, $9.95
Everything® Easy Large-Print Crosswords Book
Everything® Games Book, 2nd Ed.
Everything® Giant Book of Crosswords
Everything® Giant Sudoku Book, $9.95
Everything® Giant Word Search Book
Everything® Kakuro Challenge Book, $9.95
Everything® Large-Print Crossword Challenge Book
Everything® Large-Print Crosswords Book
Everything® Large-Print Travel Crosswords Book
Everything® Lateral Thinking Puzzles Book, $9.95
Everything® Literary Crosswords Book, $9.95
Everything® Mazes Book
Everything® Memory Booster Puzzles Book, $9.95

Everything® Movie Crosswords Book, $9.95
Everything® Music Crosswords Book, $9.95
Everything® Online Poker Book
Everything® Pencil Puzzles Book, $9.95
Everything® Poker Strategy Book
Everything® Pool & Billiards Book
Everything® Puzzles for Commuters Book, $9.95
Everything® Puzzles for Dog Lovers Book, $9.95
Everything® Sports Crosswords Book, $9.95
Everything® Test Your IQ Book, $9.95
Everything® Texas Hold 'Em Book, $9.95
Everything® Travel Crosswords Book, $9.95
Everything® Travel Mazes Book, $9.95
Everything® Travel Word Search Book, $9.95
Everything® TV Crosswords Book, $9.95
Everything® Word Games Challenge Book
Everything® Word Scramble Book
Everything® Word Search Book

HEALTH

Everything® Alzheimer's Book
Everything® Diabetes Book
Everything® First Aid Book, $9.95
Everything® Green Living Book
Everything® Health Guide to Addiction and Recovery
Everything® Health Guide to Adult Bipolar Disorder
Everything® Health Guide to Arthritis
Everything® Health Guide to Controlling Anxiety
Everything® Health Guide to Depression
Everything® Health Guide to Diabetes, 2nd Ed.
Everything® Health Guide to Fibromyalgia
Everything® Health Guide to Menopause, 2nd Ed.
Everything® Health Guide to Migraines
Everything® Health Guide to Multiple Sclerosis
Everything® Health Guide to OCD
Everything® Health Guide to PMS
Everything® Health Guide to Postpartum Care
Everything® Health Guide to Thyroid Disease
Everything® Hypnosis Book
Everything® Low Cholesterol Book
Everything® Menopause Book
Everything® Nutrition Book
Everything® Reflexology Book
Everything® Stress Management Book
Everything® Superfoods Book, $15.95

HISTORY

Everything® American Government Book
Everything® American History Book, 2nd Ed.
Everything® American Revolution Book, $15.95
Everything® Civil War Book
Everything® Freemasons Book
Everything® Irish History & Heritage Book
Everything® World War II Book, 2nd Ed.

HOBBIES

Everything® Candlemaking Book
Everything® Cartooning Book
Everything® Coin Collecting Book
Everything® Digital Photography Book, 2nd Ed.

Everything® Drawing Book
Everything® Family Tree Book, 2nd Ed.
Everything® Guide to Online Genealogy, $15.95
Everything® Knitting Book
Everything® Knots Book
Everything® Photography Book
Everything® Quilting Book
Everything® Sewing Book
Everything® Soapmaking Book, 2nd Ed.
Everything® Woodworking Book

HOME IMPROVEMENT

Everything® Feng Shui Book
Everything® Feng Shui Decluttering Book, $9.95
Everything® Fix-It Book
Everything® Green Living Book
Everything® Home Decorating Book
Everything® Home Storage Solutions Book
Everything® Homebuilding Book
Everything® Organize Your Home Book, 2nd Ed.

KIDS' BOOKS

All titles are $7.95
Everything® Fairy Tales Book, $14.95
Everything® Kids' Animal Puzzle & Activity Book
Everything® Kids' Astronomy Book
Everything® Kids' Baseball Book, 5th Ed.
Everything® Kids' Bible Trivia Book
Everything® Kids' Bugs Book
Everything® Kids' Cars and Trucks Puzzle and Activity Book
Everything® Kids' Christmas Puzzle & Activity Book
Everything® Kids' Connect the Dots
    Puzzle and Activity Book
Everything® Kids' Cookbook, 2nd Ed.
Everything® Kids' Crazy Puzzles Book
Everything® Kids' Dinosaurs Book
Everything® Kids' Dragons Puzzle and Activity Book
Everything® Kids' Environment Book $7.95
Everything® Kids' Fairies Puzzle and Activity Book
Everything® Kids' First Spanish Puzzle and Activity Book
Everything® Kids' Football Book
Everything® Kids' Geography Book
Everything® Kids' Gross Cookbook
Everything® Kids' Gross Hidden Pictures Book
Everything® Kids' Gross Jokes Book
Everything® Kids' Gross Mazes Book
Everything® Kids' Gross Puzzle & Activity Book
Everything® Kids' Halloween Puzzle & Activity Book
Everything® Kids' Hanukkah Puzzle and Activity Book
Everything® Kids' Hidden Pictures Book
Everything® Kids' Horses Book
Everything® Kids' Joke Book
Everything® Kids' Knock Knock Book
Everything® Kids' Learning French Book
Everything® Kids' Learning Spanish Book
Everything® Kids' Magical Science Experiments Book
Everything® Kids' Math Puzzles Book
Everything® Kids' Mazes Book
Everything® Kids' Money Book, 2nd Ed.
**Everything® Kids' Mummies, Pharaoh's, and Pyramids
    Puzzle and Activity Book**
Everything® Kids' Nature Book
Everything® Kids' Pirates Puzzle and Activity Book
Everything® Kids' Presidents Book
Everything® Kids' Princess Puzzle and Activity Book
Everything® Kids' Puzzle Book

Everything® Kids' Racecars Puzzle and Activity Book
Everything® Kids' Riddles & Brain Teasers Book
Everything® Kids' Science Experiments Book
Everything® Kids' Sharks Book
Everything® Kids' Soccer Book
Everything® Kids' Spelling Book
Everything® Kids' Spies Puzzle and Activity Book
Everything® Kids' States Book
Everything® Kids' Travel Activity Book
Everything® Kids' Word Search Puzzle and Activity Book

LANGUAGE

Everything® Conversational Japanese Book with CD, $19.95
Everything® French Grammar Book
Everything® French Phrase Book, $9.95
Everything® French Verb Book, $9.95
Everything® German Phrase Book, $9.95
Everything® German Practice Book with CD, $19.95
Everything® Inglés Book
Everything® Intermediate Spanish Book with CD, $19.95
Everything® Italian Phrase Book, $9.95
Everything® Italian Practice Book with CD, $19.95
Everything® Learning Brazilian Portuguese Book with CD, $19.95
Everything® Learning French Book with CD, 2nd Ed., $19.95
Everything® Learning German Book
Everything® Learning Italian Book
Everything® Learning Latin Book
Everything® Learning Russian Book with CD, $19.95
Everything® Learning Spanish Book
Everything® Learning Spanish Book with CD, 2nd Ed., $19.95
Everything® Russian Practice Book with CD, $19.95
Everything® Sign Language Book, $15.95
Everything® Spanish Grammar Book
Everything® Spanish Phrase Book, $9.95
Everything® Spanish Practice Book with CD, $19.95
Everything® Spanish Verb Book, $9.95
Everything® Speaking Mandarin Chinese Book with CD, $19.95

MUSIC

Everything® Bass Guitar Book with CD, $19.95
Everything® Drums Book with CD, $19.95
Everything® Guitar Book with CD, 2nd Ed., $19.95
Everything® Guitar Chords Book with CD, $19.95
Everything® Guitar Scales Book with CD, $19.95
Everything® Harmonica Book with CD, $15.95
Everything® Home Recording Book
Everything® Music Theory Book with CD, $19.95
Everything® Reading Music Book with CD, $19.95
Everything® Rock & Blues Guitar Book with CD, $19.95
Everything® Rock & Blues Piano Book with CD, $19.95
Everything® Rock Drums Book with CD, $19.95
Everything® Singing Book with CD, $19.95
Everything® Songwriting Book

NEW AGE

Everything® Astrology Book, 2nd Ed.
Everything® Birthday Personology Book
Everything® Celtic Wisdom Book, $15.95
Everything® Dreams Book, 2nd Ed.
Everything® Law of Attraction Book, $15.95
Everything® Love Signs Book, $9.95
Everything® Love Spells Book, $9.95
Everything® Palmistry Book
Everything® Psychic Book
Everything® Reiki Book

Everything® Sex Signs Book, $9.95
Everything® Spells & Charms Book, 2nd Ed.
Everything® Tarot Book, 2nd Ed.
Everything® Toltec Wisdom Book
Everything® Wicca & Witchcraft Book, 2nd Ed.

PARENTING

Everything® Baby Names Book, 2nd Ed.
Everything® Baby Shower Book, 2nd Ed.
Everything® Baby Sign Language Book with DVD
Everything® Baby's First Year Book
Everything® Birthing Book
Everything® Breastfeeding Book
Everything® Father-to-Be Book
Everything® Father's First Year Book
Everything® Get Ready for Baby Book, 2nd Ed.
Everything® Get Your Baby to Sleep Book, $9.95
Everything® Getting Pregnant Book
Everything® Guide to Pregnancy Over 35
Everything® Guide to Raising a One-Year-Old
Everything® Guide to Raising a Two-Year-Old
Everything® Guide to Raising Adolescent Boys
Everything® Guide to Raising Adolescent Girls
Everything® Mother's First Year Book
Everything® Parent's Guide to Childhood Illnesses
Everything® Parent's Guide to Children and Divorce
Everything® Parent's Guide to Children with ADD/ADHD
Everything® Parent's Guide to Children with Asperger's
    Syndrome
Everything® Parent's Guide to Children with Anxiety
Everything® Parent's Guide to Children with Asthma
Everything® Parent's Guide to Children with Autism
Everything® Parent's Guide to Children with Bipolar Disorder
Everything® Parent's Guide to Children with Depression
Everything® Parent's Guide to Children with Dyslexia
Everything® Parent's Guide to Children with Juvenile Diabetes
Everything® Parent's Guide to Children with OCD
Everything® Parent's Guide to Positive Discipline
Everything® Parent's Guide to Raising Boys
Everything® Parent's Guide to Raising Girls
Everything® Parent's Guide to Raising Siblings
**Everything® Parent's Guide to Raising Your
    Adopted Child**
Everything® Parent's Guide to Sensory Integration Disorder
Everything® Parent's Guide to Tantrums
Everything® Parent's Guide to the Strong-Willed Child
Everything® Parenting a Teenager Book
Everything® Potty Training Book, $9.95
Everything® Pregnancy Book, 3rd Ed.
Everything® Pregnancy Fitness Book
Everything® Pregnancy Nutrition Book
Everything® Pregnancy Organizer, 2nd Ed., $16.95
Everything® Toddler Activities Book
Everything® Toddler Book
Everything® Tween Book
Everything® Twins, Triplets, and More Book

PETS

Everything® Aquarium Book
Everything® Boxer Book
Everything® Cat Book, 2nd Ed.
Everything® Chihuahua Book
Everything® Cooking for Dogs Book
Everything® Dachshund Book
Everything® Dog Book, 2nd Ed.
Everything® Dog Grooming Book

Everything® Dog Obedience Book
Everything® Dog Owner's Organizer, $16.95
Everything® Dog Training and Tricks Book
Everything® German Shepherd Book
Everything® Golden Retriever Book
Everything® Horse Book, 2nd Ed., $15.95
Everything® Horse Care Book
Everything® Horseback Riding Book
Everything® Labrador Retriever Book
Everything® Poodle Book
Everything® Pug Book
Everything® Puppy Book
Everything® Small Dogs Book
Everything® Tropical Fish Book
Everything® Yorkshire Terrier Book

REFERENCE

Everything® American Presidents Book
Everything® Blogging Book
Everything® Build Your Vocabulary Book, $9.95
Everything® Car Care Book
Everything® Classical Mythology Book
Everything® Da Vinci Book
Everything® Einstein Book
Everything® Enneagram Book
Everything® Etiquette Book, 2nd Ed.
Everything® Family Christmas Book, $15.95
Everything® Guide to C. S. Lewis & Narnia
Everything® Guide to Divorce, 2nd Ed., $15.95
Everything® Guide to Edgar Allan Poe
Everything® Guide to Understanding Philosophy
Everything® Inventions and Patents Book
Everything® Jacqueline Kennedy Onassis Book
Everything® John F. Kennedy Book
Everything® Mafia Book
Everything® Martin Luther King Jr. Book
Everything® Pirates Book
Everything® Private Investigation Book
Everything® Psychology Book
Everything® Public Speaking Book, $9.95
Everything® Shakespeare Book, 2nd Ed.

RELIGION

Everything® Angels Book
Everything® Bible Book
Everything® Bible Study Book with CD, $19.95
Everything® Buddhism Book
Everything® Catholicism Book
Everything® Christianity Book
Everything® Gnostic Gospels Book
Everything® Hinduism Book, $15.95
Everything® History of the Bible Book
Everything® Jesus Book
Everything® Jewish History & Heritage Book
Everything® Judaism Book
Everything® Kabbalah Book
Everything® Koran Book
Everything® Mary Book
Everything® Mary Magdalene Book
Everything® Prayer Book

Everything® Saints Book, 2nd Ed.
Everything® Torah Book
Everything® Understanding Islam Book
Everything® Women of the Bible Book
Everything® World's Religions Book

SCHOOL & CAREERS

Everything® Career Tests Book
Everything® College Major Test Book
Everything® College Survival Book, 2nd Ed.
Everything® Cover Letter Book, 2nd Ed.
Everything® Filmmaking Book
Everything® Get-a-Job Book, 2nd Ed.
Everything® Guide to Being a Paralegal
Everything® Guide to Being a Personal Trainer
Everything® Guide to Being a Real Estate Agent
Everything® Guide to Being a Sales Rep
Everything® Guide to Being an Event Planner
Everything® Guide to Careers in Health Care
Everything® Guide to Careers in Law Enforcement
Everything® Guide to Government Jobs
Everything® Guide to Starting and Running a Catering Business
Everything® Guide to Starting and Running a Restaurant
Everything® Guide to Starting and Running a Retail Store
Everything® Job Interview Book, 2nd Ed.
Everything® New Nurse Book
Everything® New Teacher Book
Everything® Paying for College Book
Everything® Practice Interview Book
Everything® Resume Book, 3rd Ed.
Everything® Study Book

SELF-HELP

Everything® Body Language Book
Everything® Dating Book, 2nd Ed.
Everything® Great Sex Book
Everything® Guide to Caring for Aging Parents, $15.95
Everything® Self-Esteem Book
Everything® Self-Hypnosis Book, $9.95
Everything® Tantric Sex Book

SPORTS & FITNESS

Everything® Easy Fitness Book
Everything® Fishing Book
Everything® Guide to Weight Training, $15.95
Everything® Krav Maga for Fitness Book
Everything® Running Book, 2nd Ed.
Everything® Triathlon Training Book, $15.95

TRAVEL

Everything® Family Guide to Coastal Florida
Everything® Family Guide to Cruise Vacations
Everything® Family Guide to Hawaii
Everything® Family Guide to Las Vegas, 2nd Ed.
Everything® Family Guide to Mexico
Everything® Family Guide to New England, 2nd Ed.

Everything® Family Guide to New York City, 3rd Ed.
Everything® Family Guide to Northern California and Lake Tahoe
Everything® Family Guide to RV Travel & Campgrounds
Everything® Family Guide to the Caribbean
Everything® Family Guide to the Disneyland® Resort, California Adventure®, Universal Studios®, and the Anaheim Area, 2nd Ed.
Everything® Family Guide to the Walt Disney World Resort®, Universal Studios®, and Greater Orlando, 5th Ed.
Everything® Family Guide to Timeshares
Everything® Family Guide to Washington D.C., 2nd Ed.

WEDDINGS

Everything® Bachelorette Party Book, $9.95
Everything® Bridesmaid Book, $9.95
Everything® Destination Wedding Book
Everything® Father of the Bride Book, $9.95
Everything® Green Wedding Book, $15.95
Everything® Groom Book, $9.95
Everything® Jewish Wedding Book, 2nd Ed., $15.95
Everything® Mother of the Bride Book, $9.95
Everything® Outdoor Wedding Book
Everything® Wedding Book, 3rd Ed.
Everything® Wedding Checklist, $9.95
Everything® Wedding Etiquette Book, $9.95
Everything® Wedding Organizer, 2nd Ed., $16.95
Everything® Wedding Shower Book, $9.95
Everything® Wedding Vows Book, 3rd Ed., $9.95
Everything® Wedding Workout Book
Everything® Weddings on a Budget Book, 2nd Ed., $9.95

WRITING

Everything® Creative Writing Book
Everything® Get Published Book, 2nd Ed.
Everything® Grammar and Style Book, 2nd Ed.
Everything® Guide to Magazine Writing
Everything® Guide to Writing a Book Proposal
Everything® Guide to Writing a Novel
Everything® Guide to Writing Children's Books
Everything® Guide to Writing Copy
Everything® Guide to Writing Graphic Novels
Everything® Guide to Writing Research Papers
Everything® Guide to Writing a Romance Novel, $15.95
Everything® Improve Your Writing Book, 2nd Ed.
Everything® Writing Poetry Book

Available wherever books are sold! To order, call 800-258-0929, or visit us at *www.adamsmedia.com*.
Everything® and everything.com® are registered trademarks of F+W Publications, Inc.
Bolded titles are new additions to the series.
All Everything® books are priced at $12.95 or $14.95, unless otherwise stated. Prices subject to change without notice.